“十四五”职业教育国家规划教材

医学人文英语系列教材

医学人文英语

English for Medical Humanities

第三版（下册）

主编　杨劲松　徐　琴　刘　娅

副主编　刘　宇　黄晓彬　丁文凤　赖宁艺

编　委（按拼音排序）

陈　英	陈雨宇	丁文凤	段其伟	高　玮
黄橙橙	黄　芳	黄晓彬	晋桂清	赖宁艺
李朝东	李　丹	梁　楹	廖琳玉	刘春娴
刘　娅	刘永艳	刘　宇	罗　靖	宁　静
宁康健	彭　姝	石姝倩	唐韶凤	田　苗
王梦婕	王振宇	温群方	文瑞玲	谢婷婷
徐　琴	杨　帆	杨劲松	于恩江	张　敏
张桥英	张天一	张馨俪	张　燕	郑书耘
钟善奇	周　恩	祝海林		

复旦大学出版社

前　言

医学人文英语课程主要面向通过大学英语四级、六级考试，具备一定的医学专业英语表达能力的学生。

医学人文英语课程以现代外语教学理念为指导，以英语语言知识与应用技能、医学人文常识、学习策略为主要内容，以现代教育技术和信息技术为重点支撑，以医学人文素养培养为实践导向，在提高学生专业英语听、说、读、写、译各项技能综合运用能力的过程中提升学生医学人文素养。

通过引导学生浏览医学通识性英文网站，丰富教学资源，拓展学生自主学习空间，培养学生捕捉信息、理解信息、拓展信息的实践能力。

采用真实与半真实、典型的语言材料，通过课堂教学视、听、说各个环节输入各种语言信息，刺激学生对医学英语词汇语音听觉的识别，培养学生辨音、大意总结、内容推测、释意复述、短时记忆和速记的能力。

通过大量的口语练习和实践，尤其是医学行业真实对话情景，逐步培养和提高学生使用医学英语进行口头交际的能力，使学生能比较准确地表达思想，做到语音、语调、语法基本正确，语言运用基本得体。

运用以医学人文主题为中心的教学法，通过选择与医学行业相关的阅读文章和材料，培养医学生有效掌握语言知识和获取信息的能力。通过阅读扩充词汇量，做到能够用扎实的语法知识快速分析结构复杂的长、难句。帮助学生掌握充分的语篇知识，能在语篇层面上准确把握文章结构、段际关系和句际的逻辑关系、语体风格、行文思路、观点和态度。能够掌握各种阅读技能，运用演绎法和归纳法对文章进行各种推理、分析和判断，提升阅读速度。

通过对各种医学英语篇章的学习，了解医学篇章文体的特点；通过对比和分析汉英两种语言,掌握英汉翻译的基本理论,英汉词语、长句及各种文本的翻译技巧和英汉互译的能力。

通过句型仿写,在词义、词序、语法形式、修辞手法、文化背景等方面对比英汉两种语言的差异,帮助学生掌握词、句、篇的翻译技巧。

以医学人文为内容,通过系统地讲授英语写作基础知识,对学生进行各项与写作有关的单项训练和综合训练,培养学生英语谋篇布局习惯、观察能力和逻辑思维能力,提高学生的英语写作能力,做到文章语言清晰、流畅和达意,有一定的思想性,并具有较强的逻辑性,进而使学生具备一定的医学论文英语写作能力。

编　者

2023 年 2 月

目　录

Unit 1
Public Health

I. Info-storm **Web News on Public Health**

Read the web page. Then answer the questions orally.

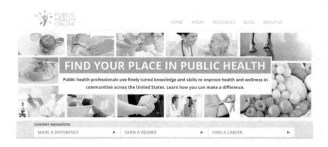

What exactly is public health? Public health is the medico-scientific study of communicable disease transmission and lifestyle-related health issues in different populations, including everything from dietary concerns in individual communities around the US to the source and progression of global pandemics. Under the umbrella of public health, government agencies, non-profits, and healthcare organizations cooperate to identify, prevent, and respond to health threats using everything from information and outreach, to vaccine deployment strategies.

While doctors diagnose and treat patients individually, public health professionals promote health on a broader scale. For example, a doctor may work with a patient to minimize the physical effects of a sexually transmitted disease (STD). A public health professional specializing in epidemiology might coordinate with community leaders to stop the spread of that very same STD. According to the Centers for Disease Control and Prevention (CDC), the nation's premier public health agency, the philosophy is simple: find out what's making people sick and killing them, and then do the things that work to protect them and make them healthier.

During the 20th century, the average lifespan worldwide increased by 30 years. Twenty-five of those can be attributed directly to advances in public health. These advances fall into three main categories: health, disease and safety.

deployment [dɪˈplɔɪmənt]	*n.* the distribution of forces in preparation for battle or work 有效运用；部署，调动
epidemiology [ˌepɪˌdiːmɪˈɒlədʒɪ]	*n.* the branch of medical science dealing with the transmission and control of disease 流行病学；传染病学
premier [ˈpremɪə(r)]	*adj.* most important，famous or successful 首要的；最著名的；最成功的；第一的
philosophy [fəˈlɒsəfɪ]	*n.* the attitude or set of ideas that guides the behaviour of a person or organization 生活[工作]准则

（1）What is the philosophy of public health?

_____

（2）Why does the average lifespan increased in the 20th century?

_____

（3）How to get a degree in public health conveniently?

_____

II. Watching-in　What Is Public Health?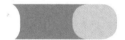

1. View the video clips. Match the photos (A – D) to the dialogues (1 – 4). Then answer the following questions.

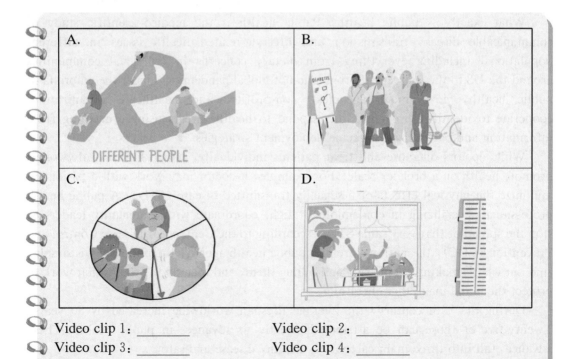

Video clip 1: _____　　Video clip 2: _____
Video clip 3: _____　　Video clip 4: _____

(1) How does public health programs improve the health of the community?

_____

(2) What kinds of measures does public health programs provide when dealing with infants disease?

_____

(3) What benefits of public health bring to the world?

_____

minimize ['mɪnɪmaɪz]	*v*. to reduce sth，especially sth bad，to the lowest possible level 使减少到最低限度
antibiotic [ˌæntɪbaɪ'ɒtɪk]	*n*. a substance，for example penicillin，that can destroy or prevent the growth of bacteria and cure infections 抗生素（如青霉素）
infectious [ɪn'fekʃəs]	*adj*. disease can be passed easily from one person to another，especially through the air they breath 传染性的,感染的（尤指通过呼吸）
sanitation [ˌsænɪ'teɪʃn]	*n*. the equipment and systems that keep places clean，especially by removing human waste 卫生设备；卫生设施体系
halt [hɔːlt]	*v*. to stop；to make sb/sth stop （使）停止,停下
strive [straɪv]	*v*. to try very hard to achieve sth 努力；奋斗；力争；力求

Unit 1　Unit 2　Unit 3　Unit 4　Unit 5　Unit 6　Unit 7　Unit 8

2. **View the video clips again. Fill in the blanks to complete the sentences which can help you get the gist of the content.**

(1)

　　Even before a child is born，a quest to 1) _____ its long and healthy life begins. All over the world，public health programs work to improve the health and 2) _____ of communities by identifying 3) _____ that affect different people in different places at different stages of life and finding the best ways to 4) _____ them. It's about giving everyone the best chance to lead long，healthy，5) _____ lives from the very beginning to the very end.

(2)

　　A child dies every three seconds from 1) _____ disease. But public health 2) _____ can prevent this by promoting things like breastfeeding，3) _____ and antibiotics. Where children die because they have no 4) _____ to safe water or basic sanitation，public health programs can make water safe and condition 5) _____.

(3)

Where research shows us who has the highest risk of developing certain conditions，public health 1) _____ it to the real world. It turns evidence into the advice and 2) _____ we need to lead active, healthy lives away from danger. It helps us make the right choices and form 3) _____ that impact on our health now and long into the future. Poor health doesn't just cost lives, it costs money, too. By preventing, detecting and treating disease as 4) _____ as we can, public health can help to 5) _____ the spiraling costs of treatment, saving lives and saving money.

(4)

Public health is about understanding the huge impact that our financial，social and environmental 1) _____ have on our health and 2) _____ the differences between us to make us all healthier. It's about making health 3) _____ in mind and body, at home and at work，by supporting 4) _____，families and communities in the environments they live and work in. It's about working to ensure that no one is left out or left behind as we 5) _____ for better. Public health，preventing disease，prolonging life，promoting health for everyone at every stage of life.

III. Leading-in　Defining Healthcare System

1. **View a video clip and fill in the blanks. Then define the term "public health" in your own words.**

— Public health is a vaccine that prevents disease.

— Public health is a (1) _____ who discovers the source of a salmonella outbreak.

— Public health is outreach that helps prevent tobacco and drug use.

— So，what is public health? While a doctor treats (2) _____，public health looks at the health of a (3) _____. We research the risk of disease and injury in a population and (4) _____ to prevent them before they occur. Our early successes helped stop the spread of infectious diseases by improving housing and (5) _____. With a greater scientific understanding of health，well-being and (6) _____，we introduced prevention and early protection activities that helped increase (7) _____ by more than 20 years.

— Public health is (8) _____ to prenatal services for healthy babies and moms.

— Public health is safety advances like (9) _____ laws that have saved millions of lives.

— Public health is access to (10) _____ and education to prevent sexually transmitted diseases.

— Public health was founded on the principle of (11) _____ . As a basic right, everyone should have the opportunity for good health. Did you know, only a small amount of what affects our health actually happens in the doctor's office. In fact, our health is mostly determined by the (12) _____ environments in which we live, learn, work and play.

2. **Read the following passage and answer these questions.**

   (1) What is the definition of public health?

   _____

   _____

   (2) What are the common public health initiatives mainly about?

   _____

   _____

   (3) Why preventive medicine should be considered the medical specialty?

   _____

   _____

   (4) What is the simple and nonmedical method to prevent diseases?

   _____

   _____

   (5) What do you think of public health program?

   _____

   _____

Passage A

What Is Public Health?

Definition

Public health has been defined as "the science and art of preventing disease, prolonging life and promoting health through the organized efforts and informed choices of society, organizations, public and private, communities and individuals". Analyzing the determinants of health of a population and the threats it faces is the basis for public health. The public can be as small as a handful of people or as large as a village or an entire city; in the case of a pandemic it may encompass several continents. The concept of health takes into account physical, psychological, and social well-being.

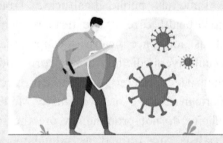

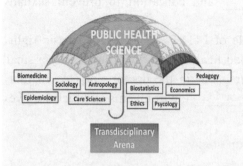

Public health is an interdisciplinary field. For example, epidemiology, biostatistics, social sciences and management of health services are all relevant. Other important subfields include environmental health, community health, behavioral health, health economics, public policy, mental health, health education, health politics, occupational safety, disability, oral health, gender issues in health, and sexual and reproductive health. Public health, together with primary care, secondary care, and tertiary care, is part of a country's overall healthcare system. Public health is implemented through the surveillance of cases and health indicators, and through the promotion of healthy behaviors. Common public health initiatives include promotion of hand-washing and breastfeeding, delivery of vaccinations, promoting ventilation and improved air quality both indoors and outdoors, suicide prevention, smoking cessation, obesity education, increasing healthcare accessibility and distribution of condoms to control the spread of sexually transmitted diseases.

Public health is related to global health which is the health of populations in the worldwide context. It has been defined as "the area of study, research and practice that places a priority on improving health and achieving equity in health for all people worldwide". International health is a field of healthcare, usually with a public health emphasis, dealing with health across regional or national boundaries. Public health is not the same as public healthcare (publicly

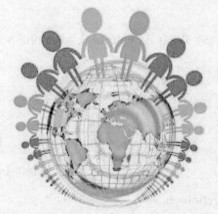

funded health care). The term preventive medicine is related to public health, such as aerospace health, occupational health, and public health and general preventative medicine. Jung, Boris and Lushniak argue that preventive medicine should be considered the medical specialty for public health but note that the American College of Preventive Medicine and American Board of Preventive Medicine do not prominently use the term "public health". Preventive medicine specialists are trained as clinicians and address complex health needs of a population such as by assessing the need for disease prevention programs, using the best methods to implement them, and assessing their effectiveness.

Since the 1990s many scholars in public health have been using the term "population health". There are no medical specialties directly related to population health. Valles argues that consideration of health equity is a fundamental part of population health. Scholars such as Coggon and Pielke express concerns about bringing general issues of wealth distribution into population health. Pielke worries about "stealth issue advocacy" in population health. Jung, Boris and Lushniak consider population health to be a concept that is the goal of an activity called public health practiced through the specialty preventive medicine.

Lifestyle medicine uses individual lifestyle modification to prevent or revert disease and can be considered a component of preventive medicine and public health. It is implemented as part of primary care rather than a specialty in its own right. Valles argues that the term "social medicine" has a narrower and more biomedical focus than the term "population health".

Public health aims are achieved through surveillance of cases and the promotion of healthy behaviors, communities and environments. Analyzing the determinants of health of a population and the threats it faces is the basis for public health.

Methods

Many diseases are preventable through simple, nonmedical methods. For example, research has shown that the simple act of handwashing with soap can prevent the spread of many contagious diseases. In other cases, treating a disease or controlling a pathogen can be vital to preventing its spread to others, either during an outbreak of infectious disease or through contamination of food or water supplies. Public health communications programs, vaccination programs and distribution

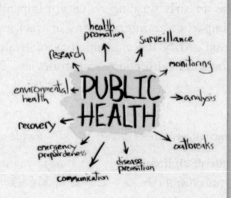

of condoms are examples of common preventive public health measures.

Public health, together with primary care, secondary care, and tertiary care, is part of a country's overall health care system. Many interventions of public health interest are delivered outside of health facilities, such as food safety surveillance, distribution of condoms and needle-exchange programs for the prevention of transmissible diseases.

Public health requires Geographic Information Systems (GIS) because risk, vulnerability and exposure involve geographic aspects.

Public Health Program

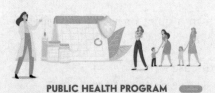

PUBLIC HEALTH PROGRAM

Most governments recognize the importance of public health programs in reducing the incidence of disease, disability, and the effects of aging and other physical and mental health conditions. However, public health generally receives significantly less government funding compared with medicine. Although the collaboration of local health and government agencies is considered best practice to improve public health, the pieces of evidence available to support this is limited. Public health programs providing vaccinations have made major progress in promoting health, including substantially reducing the occurrence of cholera and polio and eradicating smallpox, diseases that have plagued humanity for thousands of years.

Three former directors of the Global Smallpox Eradication Program reading the news that smallpox had been globally eradicated, 1980. The World Health Organization (WHO) identifies core functions of public health programs including providing leadership on matters critical to health and engaging in partnerships where joint action is needed; shaping a research agenda and stimulating the generation, translation and dissemination of valuable knowledge; setting norms and standards and promoting and monitoring their implementation; articulating ethical and evidence-based policy options; monitoring the health situation and assessing health trends. In particular, public health surveillance programs can serve as an early warning system for impending public health emergencies; document the impact of an intervention, or track progress towards specified goals; and monitor and clarify the epidemiology of health problems, allow priorities to be set, and inform health policy and strategies.

encompass [ɪnˈkʌmpəs]	*v*. awide range of ideas, subjects, etc. 包含;包括
interdisciplinary [ˌɪntəˈdɪsɪplɪnərɪ]	*adj*. involving different areas of knowledge or study 多学科的;跨学科的
behavioral [bɪˈheɪvjərəl]	*adj*. of or relating to behavior; pertaining to reactions made in response to social stimuli 行为的
tertiary [ˈtɜːʃərɪ]	*adj*. coming next after the second and just before the fourth in position 第三的,第三位的,第三级的
breastfeed [ˈbrestfiːd]	*v*. when a woman breastfeeds, she feeds her baby with milk from her breasts 用母乳喂养;哺乳
aerospace [ˈeərəʊspeɪs]	*n*. the industry of building aircraft and vehicles and equipment to be sent into space 航空航天(工业);航空航天技术
stealth [stelθ]	*n*. the fact of doing sth in a quiet or secret way 偷偷摸摸;不声张的活动;秘密行动
pathogen [ˈpæθədʒɪn]	*n*. a thing that causes disease 病原体

contagious [kən'teɪdʒəs]	*adj.* transmissible by direct or indirect contact; communicable 有传染性的
intervention [ˌɪntə'venʃən]	*n.* action taken to inprore or help a situation 介入
transmissible [trænz'mɪsəbl]	*adj.* (of disease) capable of being transmitted by infection 可传播的
involve [ɪn'vɒlv]	*v.* engage as a participant 涉及;包含
cholera ['kɒlərə]	*n.* an infectious disease of tropical countries which attacks esp. the stomach and bowels, and often leads to death 霍乱
monitor ['mɒnɪtə(r)]	*v.* to watch and check sth over a period of time in order to see how it develops 监管
implementation [ˌɪmplɪmen'teɪʃən]	*n.* the act of enforcing, carrying into effects 执行;落实

Unit 1 Unit 2 Unit 3 Unit 4 Unit 5 Unit 6 Unit 7 Unit 8

3. Match each of the terms listed below with the numbered definition. Write the letter in the space provided.

A. determinant	E. tertiary	I. revert
B. encompass	F. prominent	J. component
C. reproductive	G. distribution	K. surveillance
D. initiative	H. modification	L. vulnerability

(1) _____ : connected with reproducing babies, young animals or plants

(2) _____ : the act of carefully watching a person suspected of a crime or a place where a crime may be committed

(3) _____ : the way that sth is shared or exists over a particular area or among a particular group of people

(4) _____ : to return to the original owner again

(5) _____ : important or well known

(6) _____ : a thing that decides whether or how sth happens

(7) _____ : third in order, rank or importance

(8) _____ : to include a large number or range of things

(9) _____ : a new plan for dealing with a particular problem or for achieving a particular purpose

(10) _____ : susceptibility to injury or attack

(11) _____ : one of several parts of which sth is made

(12) _____ : the act or process of changing sth in order to improve it or make it more acceptable; a change that is made

IV. Critical Reading　Further Reading on Public Health

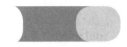

1. History of Public Health

Read the following passage and complete the exercises that follow.

A. Fill in the blanks to complete the table.

Time	
18th century	(1) _____ were used for the containment of contagious disease, which reflected (2) _____ for the control of diseases.
19th century	(3) _____ was focused on the issue of sanitation. In 1875, England carried out the Public Health Act, dealing with various (4) _____ and making a solid foundation for health system in the world.
20th century	There were some progresses in public health. The royal commission in the UK re-examined the Poor Law in 1909, which led to a proposal for a more cohesive state medical service. Recently, public health emphasize more on (5) _____ _____. Besides, (6) _____ is put as the first priority in health education.

B. Judge whether the following statements are true (T) or false (F).

_____ (1) There are two factors influenced the modern public health system: the increasing knowledge and awareness about the source and control of disease.

_____ (2) People without work cannot receive help from the government.

_____ (3) Due to expanded population size in some communities of the US, the government should carry out more formal policies to take care of the sick.

_____ (4) A new turn had taken in the 20th century.

_____ (5) America also considered an effective administrative regimen for the supervision and regulation of community health under the UK's influence.

Passage B

History of Public Health

This article presents a brief overview of the history of public health from the Middle Ages towards the present day, first beginning with a brief characterization of public health.

The development of public health began in ancient times. Health measures involved, for example, the quarantine of leprosy victims in the Middle Ages. Early international efforts in disease control occurred in national quarantines in Europe and the middle east. Over time, correlations between disease and environment were increasingly understood and refined, and from the 14th century onwards the plague epidemics spurred efforts to improve sanitation.

During the last 150 years two factors have shaped the modern public health system:

1. The proliferation of scientific knowledge about the source and control of disease

2. Increasing acceptance of disease control as possible and as a public responsibility

In England, since the late 16th century, the Poor Laws were formulated to help the deserving, but struggling, poor affected by:

- misfortune
- death of a breadwinner
- unemployment
- sickness
- inadequate wages

The level of maintenance was lowly and, sometimes, the able-bodied were required to work for their keep in a poorhouse or workhouse. Poor Law support was deemed a last resort, for otherwise, it might negate the will to work.

Medical services did not comprise a large fraction of Poor Law provision for the unfortunate, but many Poor Law Guardians hired the services of local doctors.

18th Century

By the 18th century, quarantine was commonly used for the containment of contagious disease. By this time, the right of each human being to health (and liberty and the pursuit of happiness) was brought into focus. Though the relationship between individual rights and the responsibility of the state was not always clear.

The Poor Laws were increasingly recognized as inappropriate and ineffective for the new economic circumstances of the age. In America, as the population size of specific communities expanded, more formal arrangements were required for the care of the sick. In Europe, an increasing population size coincided with a heightened awareness of infant death and of the unsavory conditions to be found in prisons and mental institutions.

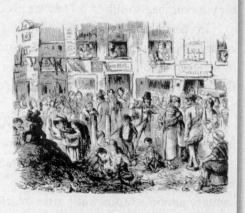

By the end of the 18th century in America, several cities including Boston and New York had established permanent measures for quarantine and isolation. These measures reflected a shift in understanding about disease from the individual, and as natural effects of the human condition, and more toward state responsibility — where the disease was potentially controllable through public action.

19th Century

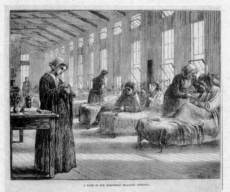

A WARD IN THE HAMPSTEAD SMALLPOX HOSPITAL.

The nineteenth century was a turning point in public health. From the 4th and 5th century BC the causal relationship between disease and the environment was established for example in the work of Hippocrates, whose book *Airs, Waters and Places* remained the theoretical framework for epidemic disease until the 19th century when the new sciences of bacteriology and immunology emerged.

The 19th century saw what has been dubbed "the great sanitary awakening" (Winslow, 1923) — where filth was identified as both a cause of disease and a mode of transmission — whereby social reforms became centered upon the issue of sanitation. Improvements in sanitary conditions occurred simultaneously in a few European countries as well as in the United States.

During the advance of the industrial revolution, the health and welfare of ordinary workers deteriorated. The increasing urbanization of populations exacerbated the occurrence of filthy environmental conditions, particularly in working-class areas, and thereby the incidence of disease. In London, for instance, smallpox, cholera, typhoid, and tuberculosis became widespread.

By the mid-nineteenth century, the hospital was a stable feature of the medical landscape. Though the limitations were that hospitals took in patients only after they succumbed to illness: They were curative rather than preventative.

In England, Edwin Chadwick (1800-1890) went beyond the known correlation between poverty and disease and argued that disease caused poverty too in his Report on the Sanitary Conditions of the Labouring Population of Great Britain (1842). Chadwick advocated for a clean system of water supply and the removal of refuge.

In England, the Public Health Act of 1875 touched housing, ventilation, sewage drainage, water supply, nuisances, dangerous trades, contagious diseases, and a plethora of other public issues thus providing the basis for the most successful health system in the world. The 1875 Act provided the standards for British sanitary administration until after World War I.

Advances in public health in England exerted a strong influence upon the US, where there was likewise a need for an effective administrative regimen for the supervision and regulation of community health. In Russia，after the communist revolution，rural medical services were massively expanded upon，to provide medical care for the entire population. The system has since inspired similar ventures in other European and Asian countries.

20th Century

The beginning of the 20th century saw further advances in community healthcare. In the United Kingdom，the royal commission reexamined the Poor Law in 1909. This led to a proposal for a more cohesive state medical service — a precursor to the 1946 National Health Service Act.

More recently，public health interests have turned to disorders such as cancer，cardiovascular disease，lung disease，and arthritis. The interrelationship between these disorders and the environment has been subject to investigation. Health education aimed at the prevention of disease became increasingly prioritized.

quarantine [ˈkwɒrəntiːn]	*n.* a period of time when an animal or a person that has or may have a disease is kept away from others in order to prevent the disease from spreading（为防传染的）隔离期；检疫
leprosy [ˈleprəsɪ]	*n.* an infectious disease that causes painful white areas on the skin and can destroy nerves and flesh 麻风
plague [pleɪg]	*n.* a quick-spreading quick-killing disease，esp. a particular one that produces high fever and swelling on the body 瘟疫（尤指鼠疫）
spur [spɜː(r)]	*v.* to encourage sb to do sth or to encourage them to try harder to achieve sth 鞭策；激励；刺激；鼓舞
sanitation [ˌsænɪˈteɪʃən]	*n.* the equipment and systems that keep places clean，especially by removing human waste 卫生设备；卫生设施体系
proliferation [prəʊˌlɪfəˈreɪʃən]	*n.* the sudden increase in the number or amount of sth；a large number of a particular thing 激增；涌现；增殖；大量的事物
deem [diːm]	*v.* keep in mind or convey as a conviction or view 认为，相信
fraction [ˈfrækʃən]	*n.* a small part or amount of sth 小部分；少量；一点儿

exacerbate [ɪgˈzæsəbeɪt]	*v*. to make sth worse，especially a disease or problem 使恶化；使加剧；使加重
filthy [ˈfɪlθɪ]	*adj*. very dirty and unpleasant 肮脏的；污秽的
tuberculosis [tjuːˌɒbɜːkjʊˈləʊsɪs]	*n*. a serious infectious disease that usu. attacks the lungs 肺结核
plethora [ˈpleθərə]	*n*. an amount that is greater than is needed or can be used 过多；过量；过剩

2. China's Great Improvement in the Quality of Medical and Health Services

Read the following passage to complete the note-taking table，and then check your understanding.

Resource factors of the medical and health-service	
Public hospital	From 2011 to 2015，there were (1) _____ , 18,000 town and township health centers, and (2) _____ and community health centers. By the end of 2016，there were (3) _____ in China.
Health personnel	The medical education system in China was (4) _____ in the world. By the end of 2016，more and more students graduated from (5) _____ , secondary schools with medical courses, and (6) _____ .
Private hospital	China spares no effort to support the development of (7) _____ in starting nonprofit medical institutions, which account for (8) _____ .
Community and rural medical conditions	China makes (9) _____ as first priority. It takes (10) _____ as the medical and health centers of the county, and places them at the core of the (11) _____ rural medical and health service network at the county, township and village levels. The result is almost every town or township has (12) _____ , every administrative village has (13) _____ , and every 1,000 rural residents have (14) _____ .
Medical and health service supply	(15) A mechanism _____ has been erected, which combines professional public health institutions, general and specialized hospitals, and community medical and health institutions. A mechanism for realizing the combination of treatment and prevention, and (16) _____ and treatment system are improving. Besides，(17) _____ are provided.
The quality and safety of medical services	Medical Quality Management Measures have been formulated，and the medical quality management and control system have been improved. The problem of (18) _____ have been completely resolved. (19) _____ covers more than 90 percent of hospitals at Grade II and above. (20) _____ have been attached great importance.

Drug supply security	Due to drug supply security system, the prices of basic drugs and drugs for hepatitis B and (21) _____ have dropped. The policy to ensure drug supply for (22) _____ have been also improved. There were 323 innovative drugs for clinical research from 2011 to 2015.
TCM	China gives TCM great support in recent years. It issued the Outline of the Strategic Plan on the Development of Traditional Chinese Medicine (2016 – 2030). Since 2011, 49 achievements in TCM scientific research have received national science and technology awards.

Passage C

China's Great Improvement in the Quality of Medical and Health Services

China is committed to improving the accessibility and convenience of medical and health resources, and the quality and efficiency of medical services at the same time. It aims to accelerate the building of an integrated medical and health service system of good quality and high efficiency, and improve the medicine supply system. More and more people are satisfied with their visits to hospitals.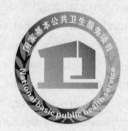

The resource factors of the medical and health-service system keep increasing. From 2011 to 2015, China invested RMB 42 billion to support the building of 1,500 county-level hospitals, 18,000 town and township health centers, and more than 100,000 village clinics and community health centers. By the end of 2016, there were 983,394 medical and health institutions in China, among which 29,140 were hospitals (12,708 public hospitals and 16,432 private ones), 36,795 town and township health centers, 34,327 community health centers (stations), 3,481 disease prevention and control centers, 2,986 health inspection institutes (centers), and 638,763 village clinics; there were also 5.291 million items of medical equipment each worth RMB 10,000 or more, among which 125,000 were worth more than RMB 1 million each. In 2016, the number of beds in medical institutions increased by 395,000 compared with 2015 — 5.37 beds for every 1,000 people; the number of beds in hospitals increased by 358,000. There were 266 hospitals of ethnic health care, with 26,484 beds, providing 9.687 million treatment sessions annually, and the number of discharged patients reached 588,000.

Health personnel optimized. China has built a medical education system of the largest scale in the world. By the end of 2016, there were 922 medical colleges and universities in China, 1,564 secondary schools with medical courses, 238 organizations granting master's degrees, and 92 granting doctoral degrees. The number of students at these schools had reached 3.95 million, among whom 1.14

million were students of clinical majors and 1.8 million of nursing majors. Fourteen educational institutions now offer specialties in ethnic healthcare, and research into ethnic healthcare in TCM majors, with about 170,000 students. TCM colleges in Yunnan, Guangxi and Guizhou offer undergraduate specialties of healthcare of the Dai, Zhuang and Miao peoples. Some ethnic-healthcare colleges and TCM colleges cooperate to cultivate personnel specializing in ethnic healthcare. By the end of 2016, the number of health workers totaled 11.173 million, with 8.454 million technical personnel, and 2.31 physicians for every 1,000 people; practicing (assistant) physicians with a college degree or above made up 81.2 percent of the total. The number of high-caliber professionals is increasing year by year. The number of nurses for every 1,000 people has reached 2.54, and the ratio of doctors to nurses has reached 1:1.1.

The nongovernmental sectors operating hospitals are growing. China supports nongovernmental sectors in starting nonprofit medical institutions, and promotes equal treatment between nonprofit private hospitals and public hospitals. We encourage physicians to make use of their spare time, and retired physicians to work in community medical and health institutions or open clinics. Private hospitals now account for more than 57 percent of all hospitals, the number of beds in medical and health institutions operated by nongovernmental sectors has increased by 81 percent compared with 2011, and their outpatient visits take up 22 percent of the total in China. Now, of the physicians who have obtained licenses that give them permission to work for more than one organization, more than 70 percent also work in medical institutions operated by nongovernmental sectors.

Community and rural medical conditions further improve. China gives priority to community and rural medical development in terms of the establishment of medical and health systems, the setting up of medical service institutions and the team building of medical service personnel. It takes county-level hospitals as the medical and health centers of the county, and places them at the core of the three-tier rural medical and health service network at the county, township and village levels. It focuses on the operation of one or two county-level hospitals (including TCM hospitals) in each county (city). Now almost every town or township has a health center, every administrative village has a village clinic, and every 1,000 rural residents have a village doctor.

Medical and health service supply is becoming more refined and targeted. China has established a mechanism for serious illness prevention and control that combines professional public health institutions, general and specialized hospitals, and community medical and health institutions. We are enhancing the mechanism for information sharing and interconnection, promoting the integrated development of chronic disease prevention, control and management, and realizing the combination of treatment and prevention. We are building a comprehensive classified diagnosis and treatment system, guiding the formation of a rational medical treatment order featuring primary treatment at the community level, two-way transfer treatment, interconnection between different levels and different treatments for acute and chronic diseases, and improving the service chain of treatment, rehabilitation and long-term care. The diagnosis and treatment rate based on appointments in Grade III hospitals has reached 38.6 percent, and nearly 400 medical institutions have set up ambulatory surgery centers. We are also providing family physician contracted services. More than 80 percent of citizens are satisfied with the skills and attitude of family physicians. The people's service experience has greatly improved.

The quality and safety level of medical services continues to rise. We have formulated Medical Quality Management Measures, gradually established and improved the medical quality management and control system, released quality control indicators, and conducted informationalized quality monitoring and feedback. We have promoted clinical pathway management (CPM) by developing 1,212 clinical pathways, which cover almost all common and frequently occurring diseases. We have released and 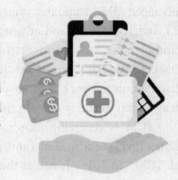 implemented the National Action Plan to Contain Antimicrobial Resistance (2016 – 2020), to resolve the problem of antimicrobial resistance in a comprehensive way. We have also strengthened supervision over prescription and drug use. In 2016, the rate of inpatients using antibacterial drugs was 37.5 percent, 21.9 percentage points lower than in 2011; the usage rate in outpatient prescriptions was 8.7 percent, a decrease of 8.5 percentage points compared with the rate in 2011. Medical liability insurance covers more than 90 percent of hospitals at Grade II and above. We attach great importance to blood safety and supply. By the end of 2015, we had realized the full coverage of nucleic acid tests in blood stations, with a blood safety level equivalent to that of developed countries. We also encourage voluntary unpaid blood donations and rational clinical use of blood. In 2016, 14 million people donated blood gratis, an increase of 6.1 percent over 2015 and almost satisfying the demand for clinical blood use. Donation has become the main source of organs for transplants.

The drug supply security system keeps improving. This system, based on the national basic drug system, has made great headway. Since the implementation of the policy, the prices of basic drugs have dropped by about 30 percent on average, and basic drugs have been sold in community-level medical and health institutions with zero markup, easing the financial burden on patients. We initiated the first round of pilot projects of national drug price negotiation, reducing the purchasing prices of drugs for hepatitis B and non-small-cell lung cancer by over 50 percent, making them the lowest in the world. By the end of 2016, the patients' expenses had been reduced by nearly RMB 100 million. We have also improved the policy that ensures drug supply for rare diseases, and increased the free supply of special drugs, for instance, drugs for the prevention and treatment of HIV/AIDS. China encourages medical and pharmaceutical innovation, launching a key project named the National New Drug Innovation Program. From 2011 to 2015, 323 innovative drugs in China were approved for clinical research, 16 innovative drugs including Icotinib Hydrochloride Tablets were approved for production, 139 new chemical generic drugs entered the market, a total of more than 600 Active Pharmaceutical Ingredients (API) and over 60 pharmaceutical companies reached the international advanced GMP standard, and a number of large medical equipment such as PET-CT and 128MSCT, and advanced implantable products including brain pacemaker, bioprosthetic valve and artificial cochlea have been approved and entered the market. We have promoted the building of a modern medical and pharmaceutical distribution network that covers both the urban and rural areas, and strengthened drug supply security at the community level and in remote areas.

TCM is receiving more support from the government. From 2013 to 2015, China invested a special fund of RMB 4.6 billion to support the capacity building of TCM. In 2016, it issued the Outline of the Strategic Plan on the Development of Traditional Chinese Medicine (2016 - 2030). The revenue generated by Chinese medicine producers each with turnover over RMB 20 million per annum reached RMB 865.3 billion in that year, accounting for about one third of the total revenue generated by all the drug producers each with turnover over RMB 20 million per annum in China. Since 2011, 49 achievements in TCM scientific research have received national science and technology awards. Artemisinin, medicines for curing acute promyelocytic leukemia and other TCM and Western medicine research findings have attracted worldwide attention.

integrated [ˈɪntɪɡreɪtɪd]	in which many different parts are closely connected and work successfully together 综合的；完整统一的
personnel [ˌpɜːsəˈnel]	*n.* the people who work for an organization or one of the armed forces (组织或军队中的)全体人员, 职员
antimicrobial [ˌæntɪmaɪˈkrəʊbɪəl]	*adj.* capable of destroying or inhibiting the growth of disease-causing microbes 抗菌的

clinical [ˈklɪnɪkəl]	*adj.* relating to a clinic or conducted in or as if in a clinic and depending on direct observation of patients 诊所的,医务室的;临床的
chronic [ˈkrɒnɪk]	*adj.* continuing for a long time;constantly recurring 慢性的
pharmaceutical [ˌfɑːməˈsuːtɪkl]	*adj.* connected with making and selling drugs and medicines 制药的;配药的;卖药的
ingredient [ɪnˈɡriːdjənt]	*n.* one of the things from which sth is made, especially one of the foods that are used together to make a particular dish 成分;(尤指烹饪)原料
cochlea [ˈkɒklɪə]	*n.* a small curved tube inside the ear, which contains a small part that sends nerve signals to the brain when sounds cause it to vibrate 耳蜗
annum [ˈænəm]	*n.* year 年
leukemia [luːˈkiːmɪə]	*n.* a type of cancer of the blood, that causes weakness and sometimes death 白血病
artemisinin [ɑːtɪˈmiːsɪnɪn]	*n.* a drug obtained from the plant genus artemisia and used to treat malaria 青蒿素

3. **Lexical chunks and sentence rewriting**

   A. **Substitute the underlined part with the words or expressions you have learned.**

   (1) Public health has been <u>named</u> as "the science and art of preventing disease, prolonging life and promoting health through the organized efforts and informed choices of society, organizations, public and private, communities and individuals". (Passage A)

   Answer:

   Public health has been _____ as "the science and art of preventing disease, prolonging life and promoting health through the organized efforts and informed choices of society, organizations, public and private, communities and individuals".

   (2) The public can be as small as a handful of people or as large as a village or an entire city; in the case of a pandemic it may <u>include</u> several continents. (Passage A)

   Answer:

   The public can be as small as a handful of people or as large as a village or an entire city; in the case of a pandemic it may _____ several continents.

   (3) Public health is <u>carried out</u> through the surveillance of cases and health indicators, and through the promotion of healthy behaviors. (Passage A)

   Answer:

   Public health is _____ through the surveillance of cases and health indicators, and through the promotion of healthy behaviors.

(4) Since the 1990s many scholars in public health have been <u>applying</u> the term population health. (Passage A)

Answer:

Since the 1990s many scholars in public health have been _____ the term population health.

B. Rewrite the following sentences using the academic expressions you have learned in the articles.

(1) Strong men were required to work for their keep in a poorhouse or workhouse.

Lexical chunks: _____

Sentence rewriting: _____

_____

(2) Health measures involved, for example, isolating of leprosy victims in the Middle Ages.

Lexical chunks: _____

Sentence rewriting: _____

_____

(3) The increasing urbanization of the population has aggravated the occurrence of bad environment.

Lexical chunks: _____

Sentence rewriting: _____

_____

(4) By the mid-nineteenth century, the hospital was a stable feature of the medical field.

Lexical chunks: _____

Sentence rewriting: _____

_____

(5) 14 million people donated blood without compensation, an increase of 6.1% over 2015, basically meeting the clinical blood demand.

Lexical chunks: _____

Sentence rewriting: _____

_____

(6) Basic drugs have been sold in community-level medical and health institutions at zero price, easing the financial burden on patients.

Lexical chunks: _____

Sentence rewriting: _____

_____

(7) We have promoted the building of a modern medical distribution network that covers both the urban and rural areas.

Lexical chunks: _____

Sentence rewriting: _____

_____

4. Bilingual translation

Put the following into Chinese or vice versa.

A. English-Chinese translation

Learn the following useful expressions by translating the sentences selected from the passage.

(1) a handful of 少数，一把

Excerpt：

The public can be as small as a handful of people or as large as a village or an entire city.

Translation：

_____

_____

(2) recognize the importance of ... in 认识到……在……的重要性

Excerpt：

Most governments recognize the importance of public health programs in reducing the incidence of disease，disability，and the effects of aging and other physical and mental health conditions.

Translation：

_____

_____

(3) be identified as 被认为……

Excerpt：

Filth was identified as both a cause of disease and a mode of transmission.

Translation：

_____

_____

(4) succumb to 抵挡不住（疾病等）

Excerpt：

Though the limitations were that hospitals took in patients only after they succumbed to illness，they were curative rather than preventative.

Translation：

_____

_____

(5) exert a strong influence upon 对……产生强烈影响

Excerpt：

Advances in public health in England exerted a strong influence upon the US.

Translation：

_____

_____

(6) be committed to 致力于

Excerpt：

China is committed to improving the accessibility and convenience of medical and health resources，and the quality and efficiency of medical services at the same time.

Translation：

_____

_____

（7）give priority to 优先考虑

Excerpt：

China gives priority to community and rural medical development in terms of the establishment of medical and health systems.

Translation：

_____

_____

B. Chinese-English translation

Put the Chinese paragraph into English.

　　健康生活方式核心要点(2023)密切关注健康生活方式、生命早期营养与慢病防控相关理论,实现了全生命周期人群的全覆盖,对"三减三健"的内容也进行了丰富和完善。健康口腔中增加了对味觉的关注,如对婴幼儿和儿童青少年人群强调了清淡口味的培养;健康骨骼中增加了肌肉、关节相关内容,如职业人群要注意舒缓肌肉紧张;关注颈腰椎和关节健康。老年人应减少骨量丢失,增加肌肉力量,也延伸了健康生活方式的涵盖内容。母乳喂养、终身学习、接种疫苗等也被纳入健康生活方式的范畴。

_____

_____

_____

_____

_____

_____

_____

_____

Ⅴ. Speaking-out　Patient's Rights and Responsibilities

1. Read and say

　　Try to answer：If you are unfortunately ill，how should you protect the rights of your own？

What Is the "Patient's Bill of Rights and Responsibilities"？

　　In 1997 a presidential commission created the Patient's Bill of Rights and Responsibilities. The Patient Bill helps ensure quality healthcare. It also protects patients and healthcare workers. They also give a way for patients to address problems with the healthcare system.

What Are a Patient's Rights?

According to the Patient Bill of Rights and Responsibilities, patients have a right to:

Accurate and easy-to-understand information about their health and healthcare providers. If patients speak another language, have a physical or mental disability or don't understand something, assistance must be provided so they can make informed healthcare decisions.

Choose providers and plans that provide access to high-quality healthcare.

Emergency services whenever and wherever needed, without prior authorization or financial penalty.

Know their treatment options and make decisions about their care. If patients cannot make their own decisions, parents, guardians, family members, or other designated individuals can represent them.

Respect and nondiscriminatory care from healthcare providers and health plan administrators.

Private and protected health information. This means that patients have the right to talk privately with a doctor and that only people involved with their healthcare can see their medical records. Patients also have the right to review and copy their medical records and ask that their records be changed if they are not correct or complete.

Complain about healthcare or anything they feel dissatisfied with such as wait times, operating hours, the conduct of healthcare personnel or the quality of healthcare facilities. Patients also have a right to a fair, fast, and objective review of any complaint against their health plan, doctors, hospitals or other healthcare personnel.

2. Watch and act

Watch a video clip. Fill in the blanks and then act it out in class.

Adam: Today I'm going to fight! Fight to improve my abdominal muscles. I'm going to exercise and let my abdominal muscle (1) _____ ...Oh, how could there be so many old people!

Narrator: In June 2019, the United Nations World Population Prospects (2) _____ that population aged over 65 has become the fastest-growing group. Currently the group accounts for about nine percent of the world population. It's estimated that by 2050 the number will go up to 16 percent. That is one out of every six people will be aged over 65. Population aging has become a (3) _____ to which China isn't immune. It's estimated that by 2020, China will have about over 255 million people aged over 60, (4) _____ 17.8 percent of its total population.

As the process of population aging continues to (5) _____ , China's elderly care system reform is facing increasingly tougher challenges, such as an (6) _____ elderly care system structure. Faced with challenges, China's elderly care service market reform is (7) _____ speed. Since 2019, a dozen of provinces and municipalities, including Beijing, Shanghai and Jiangsu, have announced the revoking of permits for setting up elderly

care institutes. Elderly care institutes are becoming privatized and （8）
_____. Statistics show that up until 2017，China's privately run elderly
care institutes account for about 44 percent of the total number. With （9）
_____ as the basis，supported by communities and supplemented by
institutes，an elderly care system combining medical and elderly care is
taking shape.

Adam： What's that my ears hear? Hark! It'd be KTV. Rock "n" roll!
... *Hǎobàng*!

Narrator： The continuous improvement of its people's life quality to match the speed
of population aging is a （10）_____ of the Chinese government to ensure
the well-being of its people. In 2019，China proposes the Healthy China
2030 Strategy，which includes the elderly care system，health care system
and fitness for all. By taking the （11）_____ against population aging，
all the elderly will be able to receive care and support and feel happy and
secure.

Adam： I'm in the middle of the "time （12）_____" between childhood and old
age. I've seen the fulfilling lives of the elderly. How I wish I could live like
this when I am old.

Ⅵ. Pros/Cons   Celebrities in Healthcare System

1. Read the following passage with ten statements attached to it. Each statement contains
information given in one of the paragraphs. Identify the paragraph from which the
information is derived. Each paragraph is marked with a letter.

_____ （1）She was trained as a nurse in Germany in 1851.

_____ （2）She went to the nursing school at 33 years old and successfully
graduated with three other classmates.

_____ （3）Her work mainly involved pediatric nursing and pediatric nursing
education.

_____ （4）She cofounded the National Association of Colored Graduate Nurses.

_____ （5）Her work raised nursing to a professional level.

_____ （6）She introduced nurse-midwifery to America.

_____ （7）She was the first African-American woman to become a registered
nurse.

_____ （8）The curriculum of the school she founded laid the groundwork for
modern nursing education.

_____ （9）The nursing school she attended admitted black nursing candidates due
to her achievements.

_____ （10）She founded the Frontier Nursing Service，a team of nurse-midwives.

A) There was a time in America that nursing duties fell to nuns, or — during wars — to the military. Before the end of the 19th century, most nurses didn't have any formal training — and many lacked any education at all. Nurses were typically women who provided the sick, injured and wounded with comfort, but not necessarily good — or any — medical care. It wasn't until the extraordinary women and men on the list advocated for change and pioneered a path for nurses from bedpan to bachelor's degree that the seeds of modern nursing were born.

Florence Nightingale

B) She's been called "The Lady with the Lamp", "The Queen of Nurses" and "The Soldiers' Friend". Florence Nightingale is possibly the most well-known nurse in history.

C) Nightingale was born into a wealthy British family in 1820. She heard the call to nursing early in her life, and completed her training at the Institute of Protestant Deaconesses at Kaiserswerth in Germany in 1851. But it was what she experienced during the Crimean War that changed her path from 19th century nurse to legendary nurse.

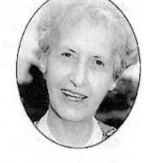

D) Upon her arrival on the scene in Turkey with a team of 38 nurses, Nightingale found devastating conditions: unsanitary hospitals, few or no supplies, and poor patient care. Nightingale and her nurses tended to the wounded British soldiers, many of whom were also sick with cholera and malaria, and set about improving hospital hygiene in an effort to reduce infections. It worked, and after the war, in 1860, she founded the Nightingale School of Nursing at St. Thomas' Hospital in London, where nursing students would learn not only about patient care, but also about the importance of good hygiene and sanitary conditions in medicine. The school's curriculum laid the groundwork for modern nursing education.

Florence Guinness Blake

E) Florence Guinness Blake was a 20th century pioneer in nursing education, advocating for better training for nurses. Blake's contributions to medical training and education helped elevate caring for patients to a professional level.

F) Blake had a special interest in caring for children, and dedicated much of her work to pediatric nursing and pediatric nursing education. She taught in the field and went on to found and oversee an advanced pediatric nursing graduate program at the University of Chicago, the first of its kind in the United States. In addition to teaching, she also wrote, edited and contributed to nursing textbooks. In the 1950s, she penned and published *The Child, His Parents and the Nurse*, a book designed to explain the parent-child relationship from infancy through adolescence, as well as address her belief that parents should be involved in the medical care of their children — concepts that are still a central part of nursing and nurse education today.

Mary Ezra Mahoney

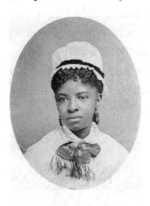

G）Mary Ezra Mahoney was the first African-American woman to complete nursing training and become a registered nurse.

H）Mahoney worked at the New England Hospital for Women and Children before she was accepted to the hospital's nursing school at the age of 33. Out of 42 candidates, only four graduated; Mahoney was one of those four.

I）Upon graduating, Mahoney registered with the Nurses' Directory at the Massachusetts Medical Library and went into private practice in New England. Because of her success, the nursing school she attended loosened their policies against admitting black nursing candidates.

J）In the face of discrimination against black nurses, Mahoney advocated for the rights of all black nurses and went on to cofound the National Association of Colored Graduate Nurses（NACGN）in 1908.

Mary Breckinridge

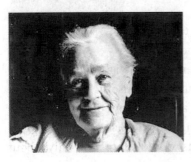

K）Mary Breckinridge dedicated her life to rural public healthcare, but it wasn't until after she suffered a series of personal tragedies, including the deaths of her two young children, that she heard the call to nursing.

L）She studied at St. Luke's Hospital in New York, and became a registered nurse in 1910. Nursing took her to Boston and Washington, D.C., and even to France as part of the American Committee for Devastated France after World War I. While in France, Breckinridge was introduced to French and British nurse-midwives, a path Breckinridge decided dovetailed perfectly with her desire to bring healthcare to rural poor families in America. When she was in her early 40s, Breckinridge studied midwifery in London and is credited with introducing nurse-midwifery to America.

M）In 1925, Breckinridge founded the Frontier Nursing Service（FNS）, a team of nurse-midwives devoted to bringing general and maternal care（including prenatal and postnatal care）to people living in the Appalachian Mountains of eastern Kentucky. The FNS nurses traveled by horseback to deliver babies and provide family care, accepting little money（or barter）as payment.

2. **Read the following statements. Decide to what extent you agree or disagree with each statement, and write your own pros or cons in the box, then set out your rational viewpoint and the reasons.**

    （1）Governments should give priority to health care in terms of people's health.

    （2）Health care is a professional field which is closely related to human health and is crucial to safeguarding people's medical needs and improving overall health.

(3) As the aging of the population intensifies, the healthcare profession will face more needs for the treatment and care of geriatric diseases.

(4) Healthcare professionals need to continuously improve their medical knowledge, communication and coordination skills, as well as leadership and management skills.

(5) Healthcare professionals have slim chances of finding employment in areas such as medical institutions, government health departments and insurance agencies.

Pros	Cons

VII. Outcome　Sentence Analysis and Essay Writing

1. Sentence-structure analysis

Analyze the following sentences and draw a tree-structure.

(1) International health is a field of healthcare, usually with a public health emphasis, dealing with health across regional or national boundaries.

(2) Preventive medicine specialists are trained as clinicians and address complex health needs of a population such as by assessing the need for disease prevention programs, using the best methods to implement them, and assessing their effectiveness.

(3) Over time, correlations between disease and environment were increasingly understood and refined, and from the 14th century onwards the plague epidemics spurred efforts to improve sanitation.

(4) From the 4th and 5th century BC the causal relationship between disease and the environment was established for example in the work of Hippocrates, whose book *Airs, Waters and Places* remained the theoretical framework for epidemic disease until the 19th century when the new sciences of bacteriology and immunology emerged.

(5) The 19th Century saw what has been dubbed "the great sanitary awakening" (Winslow, 1923) — where filth was identified as both a cause of disease and a mode of transmission — whereby social reforms became centered upon the issue of sanitation.

(6) In England, Edwin Chadwick (1800 – 1890) went beyond the known correlation between poverty and disease and argued that disease caused poverty too in his Report on the Sanitary Conditions of the Labouring Population of Great Britain (1842).

(7) Since the implementation of the policy, the prices of basic drugs have dropped by about 30 percent on average, and basic drugs have been sold in community-level medical and health institutions with zero markup, easing the financial burden on patients.

(8) The revenue generated by Chinese medicine producers each with turnover over RMB 20 million per annum reached RMB 865.3 billion in that year, accounting for about one third of the total revenue generated by all the drug producers each with turnover over RMB 20 million per annum in China.

2. Essay writing

Write an essay based on the following words.

Public health is important because it helps to prolong life. By preventing health problems, individuals can spend more of their years in good health. What do you think of your responsibility for public health? Write an essay in no less than 200 words.

_____
_____
_____
_____
_____
_____
_____
_____
_____
_____
_____
_____
_____
_____
_____

Unit 2
HIV/AIDS

Read the web page. Then answer the questions orally.

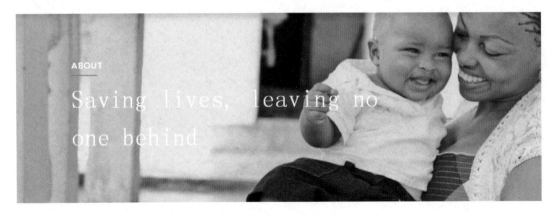

Q SEARCH | ENGLISH FRANÇ

⊕UNAIDS   WHO WE ARE   WHAT WE DO   PROGRAMME AREAS   WHERE WE WORK   RESOURCES

ABOUT

Saving lives, leaving no one behind

UNAIDS is leading the global effort to end AIDS as a public health threat by 2030 as part of the Sustainable Development Goals.

Since the first cases of HIV were reported more than 35 years ago, 78 million people have become infected with HIV and 35 million have died from AIDS-related illnesses. Since it started operations in 1996, UNAIDS has led and inspired global, regional, national and local leadership, innovation and partnership to ultimately consign HIV to history.

UNAIDS is a problem-solver. It places people living with HIV and people affected by the virus at the decision-making table and at the centre of designing, delivering and monitoring the AIDS response. It charts paths for countries and communities to get on the fast track to ending AIDS and is a bold advocate for addressing the legal and policy barriers to the AIDS response.

UNAIDS provides the strategic direction，advocacy，coordination and technical support needed to catalyse and connect leadership from governments，the private sector and communities to deliver life-saving HIV services. Without UNAIDS，there would be no strategic vision for the AIDS response.

UNAIDS is a model for United Nations reform and is the only cosponsored joint programme in the United Nations system. It draws on the experience and expertise of 11 United Nations system cosponsors and is the only United Nations entity with civil society represented on its governing body.

The UNAIDS Secretariat has offices in 70 countries，with 70% of its staff based in the field，and has a budget of US $140 million for 2018. The budget for the joint programme for 2018 is US $242 million.

inspire [ɪnˈspaɪə(r)]	*v*. to encourage sb by making them feel confident and eager to do sth 鼓舞；激励
consign [kənˈsaɪn]	*v*. give over to another for care or safekeeping, commit forever（为摆脱而）把……置于；打发；发落
bold [bəʊld]	*adj*. fearless and daring 大胆自信的；敢于冒险的
advocate [ˈædvəkeɪt]	*n*. a person who pleads for a cause or propounds an idea 拥护者；支持者
catalyse [ˈkætəlaɪz]	*v*. cause can action or process to begin 促成

（1）What is the web page mainly about?

_____

（2）How do you think about the society's view about HIV carrier?

_____

（3）Is there anything you think you can do to help people with HIV?

_____

（4）What do you think the society should do towards HIV?

_____

（5）Should government invest money on HIV prevention?

_____

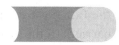

II. Watching-in   Briefing on HIV

1. **View the video clips. Match the photos (A – D) to the dialogues (1 – 4). Then answer the following questions.**

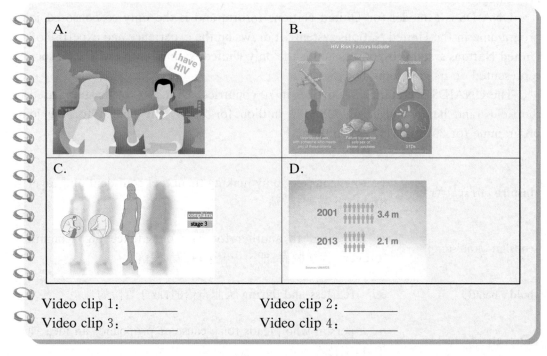

Video clip 1: _____   Video clip 2: _____

Video clip 3: _____   Video clip 4: _____

(1) What advances have been made in the treatment of HIV?

_____

(2) Who should get tested for HIV?

_____

(3) What are the key symptoms of each stage of HIV infection?

_____

2. **View the video clips again. Fill in the blanks to complete the sentences which can help you get the gist of the content.**

(1)	(2)
HIV, or Human Immunodeficiency Virus, was first recognized in the early 80s in the US, but it has its 1) _____ in 1920s Kinshasa, a bustling city more than a million pass-through each year. Thanks to newly	Anyone can be infected with HIV, regardless of age, gender or 1) _____. However, some individuals may be at greater 2) _____ and should be tested for HIV, including anyone who has used

built railways in a 2) _____ sex trade, the virus spreads up the river to Kisaeng Gani, to the diamond capital Abuja Mahi and the copper mines of Lubin Bashi, to the US in 1968 before 3) _____ around the world in the 1980s. 78 million people infected worldwide and counting, and the spread is far from 4) _____. 70% live in sub-Saharan Africa. But antiretroviral drugs offer a hope. New infections are down by over a third, mother-to-child transmission has more than 5) _____ and globally there's been a 35 percent 6) _____ in deaths. But in the Middle East and North Africa, deaths have doubled and globally only 37 percent of those living with HIV 7) _____ treatment. So, the 8) _____ now is to make those life-saving drugs available to everyone.

or shared needles for 3) _____ such as heroin, anyone who has been diagnosed with or treated for illnesses such as 4) _____, tuberculosis or TB, or a sexually 5) _____ disease or STD, anyone who has had unprotected sex. This includes cases where 6) _____ usage failed due to breaking or falling off. Testing should also be performed if unprotected sex has occurred with someone who meets any of the above 7) _____. HIV cannot be 8) _____ through symptoms since symptoms may be related to other illnesses. The only way to know if you have HIV is to take an HIV test.

(3)

An HIV infection passes through four stages. In the first stage, the body can show signs of disease like 1) _____ and swollen glands while some people who are infected remain asymptomatic in their first stage. In the second stage, recurring 2) _____, skin, mouth, and genital lesions often occur. In the third stage, you may have complaints like prolonged 3) _____, excessive 4) _____, tuberculosis in the lungs and other serious infections like meningitis. Finally, besides serious infections, the 5) _____ may be affected in the fourth stage,

(4)

There's no 1) _____ for HIV, but it can be controlled with treatment, and people with HIV can live long, healthy lives. If you're diagnosed with HIV, get started on treatment 2) _____. If you take your HIV medication as 3) _____, the amount of HIV in your blood or your viral load can become so low that a test can't 4) _____ it. This is called being undetectable. Getting and keeping an undetectable viral load can keep you healthy. Also it means you effectively have no risk of 5) _____ HIV to a partner through sex. If you're pregnant, having which can result in 6) _____ or AIDS-related 7) _____ . It may take five to fifteen years before you know that you've got AIDS. This is because sometimes it takes longer for 8) _____ to occur.

an undetectable viral load will greatly reduce the 6) _____ HIV to your baby. It's important to tell your partner that you have HIV. You and your partner may want to consider additional 7) _____ , like condoms, medicine to prevent getting HIV and making decisions that are right for both of you. Finally, talk to someone with HIV, find a 8) _____ and learn about services in your area to help you get in care, stay in care and live well.

hepatitis [ˌhepəˈtaɪtɪs]	*n.* a serious disease of the liver. There are three main forms: hepatitis A (the least serious, caused by infected food), hepatitis B and hepatitis C (both very serious and caused by infected blood). 肝炎
condom [ˈkɒndəm]	*n.* a thin rubber covering that a man wears over his penis during sex to stop a woman from becoming pregnant or to protect against disease 避孕套
genital [ˈdʒenɪtəl]	*adj.* connected with the outer sexual organs of a person or an animal 生殖的;生殖器官的
lesion [ˈliːʒən]	*n.* damage to the skin or part of the body caused by injury or by illness (因伤病导致皮肤或器官的)损伤,损害
dementia [dɪˈmenʃə]	*n.* a serious mental disorder caused by brain disease or injury, that affects the ability to think, remember and behave normally 痴呆;精神错乱
medication [ˌmedɪˈkeɪʃən]	*n.* a drug or another form of medicine that you take to prevent or to treat an illness 药;药物

1. **View a video clip and fill in the blanks. Then define the terms "HIV" and "AIDS" in your own words.**

    The human immunodeficiency virus, or HIV, is a retrovirus that (1) _____ itself within the bloodstream. After contracting HIV through certain bodily (2) _____, the body's immune system engages in a (3) _____ with the virus. As HIV circulates through the bloodstream, it attaches to some cells and repurposes them to product more virus. Using the host cell (4) _____, the virus creates new HIV. In a process called budding, the (5) _____ virus is released into the bloodstream where it (6) _____ and can infect other cells. As the replicated virus continues to spread throughout the bloodstream, it begins to (7) _____ the body's immune system, destroying white blood cells known as T cells, which are an (8) _____ part of the immune system.

2. **Read the following passage and answer these questions.**

    (1) What is the relationship between HIV and AIDS?

    _____

    _____

    (2) How does the HIV virus attack the human body?

    _____

    _____

    (3) What are the symptoms in the early stage of HIV infection?

    _____

    _____

    (4) Why can't we rely on the symptoms to tell whether someone has HIV or not?

    _____

    _____

    (5) At what stage can people with HIV transmit the virus to other people?

    _____

    _____

Passage A

An Introduction to HIV/AIDS

Human Immunodeficiency Virus (HIV)

HIV stands for human immunodeficiency virus. If left untreated, HIV can lead to the disease AIDS (acquired immunodeficiency syndrome). Unlike some other viruses, the human body can't get rid of HIV completely. So once you have HIV, you have it for life.

HIV attacks the body's immune system, specifically the CD4 cells (T cells), which help the immune system fight off infections. If left untreated, HIV reduces the number of CD4 cells in the body, making the person more likely to get infections or infection-related cancers. Over time, HIV can destroy so many of these cells that the body can't fight off infections and disease. These opportunistic infections or cancers take advantage of a very weak immune system and signal that the person has AIDS, the last state of HIV infection.

No effective cure for HIV currently exists, but with proper treatment and medical care, HIV can be controlled. The medicine used to treat HIV is called antiretroviral therapy or ART. If taken the right way, every day, this medicine can dramatically prolong the lives of many people with HIV, keep them healthy, and greatly lower their chance of transmitting the virus to others. Today, a person who is diagnosed with HIV, treated before the disease is far advanced, and stays on treatment can live nearly as long as someone who does not have HIV.

The only way to know for sure if you have HIV is to get tested. Testing is relatively simple. You can ask your healthcare provider for an HIV test. Many medical clinics, substance abuse programs, community health centers, and hospitals offer them too. You can also buy a home testing kit at a pharmacy or online.

Acquired Immunodeficiency Syndrome (AIDS)

AIDS stands for acquired immunodeficiency syndrome. AIDS is the final stage of HIV infection, and not everyone who has HIV advances to this stage.

AIDS is the stage of infection that occurs when your immune system is badly damaged and you become vulnerable to opportunistic infections. When the number of your CD4 cells falls below 200 cells per cubic millimeter of blood (200 cells/mm^3), you are considered to have progressed to AIDS. (The CD4 count of an uninfected adult/adolescent who is generally in good health ranges from 500 cells/mm^3 to 1,600 cells/mm^3.) You can also be diagnosed with AIDS if you develop one or more opportunistic infections, regardless of your CD4 count.

Without treatment, people who are diagnosed with AIDS typically survive about 3 years. Once someone has a dangerous opportunistic illness, life expectancy without treatment falls to about 1 year. People with AIDS need medical treatment to prevent death.

Stages and Symptoms of HIV Infection

The symptoms of HIV vary, depending on the individual and what stage of the disease you are in: the early stage, the clinical latency stage, or AIDS (the late stage of HIV infection). Below are the symptoms that some individuals may experience in these three stages. Not all individuals will experience these symptoms.

Early Stage of HIV

Some people infected with HIV are asymptomatic at first. Most people experience symptoms in the first month or two after becoming infected. That's because your immune system is reacting to the virus as it rapidly reproduces.

This early stage is called acute stage. Symptoms are similar to those of the flu and may last anywhere from a few days to several weeks. About 40%–90% of people have flu-like symptoms within 2–4 weeks after HIV infection. Other people do not feel sick at all during this stage, which is also known as acute HIV infection. Early infection is defined as HIV infection in the past six months (recent) and includes acute (very recent) infections. Flu-like symptoms can include:

1. Fever
2. Chills
3. Rash
4. Night sweats
5. Muscle aches
6. Sore throat
7. Fatigue
8. Swollen lymph nodes
9. Mouth ulcers

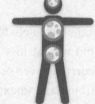

You can't rely ON SYMPTOMS to tell if you have HIV.

The only way to know for sure is to

GET TESTED

During the first few months of infection, an HIV test may provide a false-negative result. This is because it takes time for the immune system to build up enough antibodies to be detected in a blood test. But the virus is active and highly contagious during this time.

You should not assume you have HIV just because you have any of these symptoms. Each of these symptoms can be caused by other illnesses. And some people who have HIV do not show any symptoms at all for 10 years or more.

If you think you've been exposed to HIV,

GET TESTED
AS SOON AS POSSIBLE!

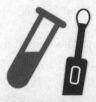

After you get tested, it's important to find out the result of your test. If you're HIV-positive, you should see a doctor and start HIV treatment as soon as possible. You are at high risk of transmitting HIV to others during the early stage of HIV infection, even if you have no symptoms. For this reason, it is very important to take steps to reduce your risk of transmission. If you're HIV-negative, explore HIV-prevention options, like pre-exposure prophylaxis (PrEP), that can help you stay negative.

Clinical Latency Stage

After the early stage of HIV infection, the disease moves into a stage called the clinical latency stage (also called "chronic HIV infection"). During this stage,

HIV is still active but reproduces at very low levels. People with chronic HIV infection may not have any HIV-related symptoms, or only mild ones.

For people who aren't taking medicine to treat HIV（called antiretroviral therapy or ART）, this period can last a decade or longer, but some may progress through this phase faster. People who are taking medicine to treat HIV, and who take their medications right way, every day, may be in this stage for several decades because treatment helps keep the virus in check.

It's important to remember that people can still transmit HIV to others during this phase even if they have no symptoms, although people who are on ART and stay virally suppressed（having a very low level of virus in their blood）are much less likely to transmit HIV than those who are not virally suppressed.

Progression to AIDS

If you have HIV and you are not on ART, eventually the virus will weaken your body's immune system and you will progress to AIDS, the late stage of HIV infection.

Symptoms can include:

1. Rapid weight loss
2. Recurring fever or profuse night sweats
3. Extreme and unexplained tiredness
4. Prolonged swelling of the lymph glands in the armpits, groin, or neck
5. Diarrhea that lasts for more than a week
6. Sores of the mouth, anus, or genitals
7. Pneumonia
8. Red, brown, pink, or purplish blotches on or under the skin or inside the mouth, nose, or eyelids
9. Memory loss, depression, and other neurologic disorders

Each of these symptoms can also be related to other illnesses. Many of the severe symptoms and illnesses of HIV disease come from the opportunistic infections that occur because your body's immune system has been damaged.

syndrome [ˈsɪndrəʊm]	*n.* a set of physical conditions that show sb has a particular disease or medical problem 综合征
opportunistic [ˌɒpətjuːˈnɪstɪk]	*adj.* harmful to people whose immune system has been made weak by disease or drugs 机会致病性的（对免疫系统差的人有害）
antiretroviral [ˈæntɪˌretrəʊˈvaɪrəl]	*adj.* inhibiting the process by which a retrovirus replicates 抗逆转录病毒的

therapy [ˈθerəpɪ]	*n.* the act of caring for sb (as by medication or remedial training, etc.) 疗法
cubic [ˈkjuːbɪk]	*adj.* having the form of a cube; cubical 立方的
millimeter [ˈmɪlɪˌmiːtə(r)]	*n.* a metric unit of length equal to one thousandth of a meter 毫米
expectancy [ɪkˈspektənsɪ]	*n.* the state of being expected 期望值
latency [ˈleɪtənsɪ]	*n.* the state or quality of being latent 潜伏
asymptomatic [ˌeɪsɪmptəˈmætɪk]	*adj.* neither causing nor exhibiting symptoms of disease 无症状的
acute [əˈkjuːt]	*adj.* reacting readily to stimuli or impressions; sensitive 急性的
swollen lymph nodes	淋巴结肿
negative [ˈnegətɪv]	*n.* expressing or consisting of a negation or refusal or denial 阴性的
antibody [ˈæntɪˌbɒdɪ]	*n.* a substance that the body produces in the blood to fight disease, or as a reaction when certain substances are put into the body 抗体
positive [ˈpɒzətɪv]	*adj.* showing clear evidence that a particular substance or medical condition is present 阳性的；证明……存在的
pre-exposure prophylaxis [ˌprɒfɪˈlæksɪs]	接触前预防
in check	受控制的
suppressed [səˈprest]	*adj.* kept from growing, developing or continuing 被抑制的
profuse [prəʊˈfjuːs]	*adj.* plentiful; copious 丰富的
armpit [ˈɑːmpɪt]	*n.* the hollow under the upper part of the arm at the shoulder 腋窝
groin [grɔɪn]	*n.* the crease or hollow at the junction of the inner part of each thigh with the trunk, together with the adjacent region and often including the external genitals 腹股沟
diarrhea [ˌdaɪəˈrɪə]	*n.* excessive and frequent evacuation of watery feces 腹泻，痢疾

anus ['eɪnəs]	*n.* the opening at the lower end of the digestive tract through which solid waste is eliminated from the body 肛门
pneumonia [njuː'məunɪə]	*n.* a serious illness affecting one or both lungs that makes breathing difficult 肺炎
blotch [blɒtʃ]	*n.* a mark, usually not regular in shape, on skin, plants, material（皮肤、植物、物体等上面不规则的）斑点
neurologic [ˌnjuərə'lɒdʒɪk]	*adj.* of or relating to or used in or practicing neurology 神经（病）学的

3. **Match each of the terms listed below with the numbered definition. Write the letter in the space provided.**

A. immunity	E. diagnose	I. opportunistic
B. antiretroviral	F. prolong	J. testing kit
C. expectancy	G. prevention	K. therapy
D. syndrome	H. mutate	L. immunodeficiency

(1) _____ : to find out what illness someone has, or what the cause of a fault is, after doing tests, examinations, etc.

(2) _____ : harmful to people whose immune system has been made weak by disease or drugs

(3) _____ : the state of being immune to a disease

(4) _____ : to change and develop a new form

(5) _____ : the act of preventing

(6) _____ : to deliberately make something last longer

(7) _____ : inhibiting the process by which a retrovirus replicates

(8) _____ : the treatment of an illness or injury over a fairly long period of time

(9) _____ : a weakness in a person's immune system or the failure of a person's immune system

(10) _____ : an illness which consists of a set of physical or mental problems — often used in the name of illnesses

(11) _____ : a set of tools, equipment etc. for test

(12) _____ : the feeling or hope that something exciting, interesting, or good is about to happen

Further Reading on HIV and AIDS

1. HIV and AIDS: An Origin Story

Read the following passage and fill in the blanks to complete the table.

Year	
1970s	When HIV first began infecting humans in the 1970s, scientists were unaware of its existence.
1980s	**Situation** Due to emergence of (1) _____, scientists began to connect the dots between these new diagnoses, plus a number of other opportunistic infections in 1981, when they found (2) _____ HIV.
	Public policy responds In America, the (3) _____ were instituted; the FDA began to consider whether the nation's supply of (4) _____ was safe. The concept of (5) _____ was first introduced to the global populace. At the end of 1986 and the beginning of 1987, Azidothymidine (AZT), the first drug to prove effective against the rapidly replicating HIV virus, was put on (6) __ _____ .
1990s	**Situation** During 1990s, there were a growing number of people infected HIV in various countries. **Research and policy breakthroughs** There were researches gaining progress. ACTG 076 was effective in (7) _____ _____ , and Saquinavir was approved by the FDA in record time. While significant breakthroughs have made in (8) _____, due to the efforts of CDC, (9) _____ had a significant increase, and HIV/AIDS education gradually stepped into the schools in America. Internationally, the WHO AIDS program was replaced by the UNAIDS Global Programme that is still in existence today. **However, the situation in Africa was grim.** Because some African politicians refused to acknowledge (10) _____ between men, the nation's homosexual population was in a health crisis. Additionally, there was a lack of (11) _____ , which made it difficult to administrate medications that might have slowed the rate of HIV infection in these countries.
2000 – today	Since 2000, there were new risk of new infection of HIV, owning to the rise of (12) _____ in Asia. While in 2010, the WHO released a report of examing HIV and AIDS in its 25-year history. It demonstrated that the rate of (13) _____ was stable in US, and had slowed down in other developed countries, because of public awareness campaigns about (14) _____ and other methods of transmission. Besides, even though the "3 by 5 Plan" carried out by WHO for African people failed, it had been (15) _____ to deliver care to sub-Saharan Africans by 2010.

Passage B

HIV and AIDS: An Origin Story

When HIV first began infecting humans in the 1970s, scientists were unaware of its existence. Now, more than 35 million people across the globe live with HIV/AIDS. The medical community, politicians and support organizations have made incredible progress in the fight against this formerly unknown and heavily stigmatized virus. Infection rates have fallen or stabilized in many countries across the world, but we have a long way to go.

1980s

Beginning in the early 1980s, new and unusual diagnostic patterns began to emerge in different parts of the world. A benign, fairly harmless cancer called Kaposi's Sarcoma, common among the elderly, started appearing as a virulent strain in younger patients. Simultaneously, a rare, aggressive form of pneumonia began to crop up with alarming frequency in another group of patients. This pneumonia sometimes evolved into a chronic condition, which was something specialists had never seen.

By 1981, scientists had begun to connect the dots between these new diagnoses, plus a number of other opportunistic infections. By the end of the year, the first case of HIV's full-blown disease state, Acquired Immunodeficiency Syndrome (AIDS), was documented.

Public policy responds

As scientists closed in on the source of this illness, public policymakers in America reacted to the epidemic. Bathhouses and clubs catering to gay clientele were closed down, and law enforcement personnel were issued gloves and masks to protect them against potential exposure. The first needle exchange programs were instituted; the FDA began to consider whether the nation's supply of banked blood was safe. The concept of "safe sex", now considered standard behavior, was first introduced to the global populace.

In late 1983, the global presence of the mysterious virus motivated European authorities and the WHO to classify the growing number of diagnoses as an epidemic. In addition to the outbreak in the US, patients with similar symptoms were documented in 15 European countries, 7 Latin American countries, Canada, Zaire (now the Democratic Republic of Congo), Haiti, Australia and Japan. Of particular concern was an outbreak in central Africa among heterosexual patients. In the US, the mortality rate approached 100%. The first annual international AIDS meetings were held in 1985.

At the end of 1986 and the beginning of 1987, the FDA administered a clinical trial of Azidothymidine (AZT), the first drug to prove effective against the rapidly replicating HIV virus. Originally a chemotherapy drug, AZT worked so well during its trial that the FDA halted the trial on the grounds that it would be unethical to deprive those patients who received a placebo of the actual drug.

1990s

By 1993, over 2.5 million cases of HIV/AIDS had been confirmed worldwide. By 1995, AIDS was the leading cause of death for Americans age 25 to 44. Elsewhere, new cases of AIDS were stacking up in Russia, Ukraine, and other parts of Eastern Europe. Vietnam, Cambodia and China also reported steady increases in cases. The UN estimated that in 1996 alone, 3 million new infections were recorded in patients under age 25.

Countless deaths in the US entertainment industry, the arts and among professional athletes deeply affected these communities — and the rate of death would not slow significantly until 1997. During this time, the US government enacted legislation that directly affected HIV-positive people. These individuals were legally prohibited from working in healthcare, donating blood, entering the country on a travel visa, or emigrating.

Research and policy breakthroughs

Meanwhile, research scientists were gaining ground. The course of infection was better understood, and the clinical definition of HIV and AIDS was refined. Other drugs went into trial, with mixed success. A drug known as ACTG 076 showed particular promise in mother-to-infant transmissions, and a drug called Saquinavir was approved by the FDA in record time. Viramune followed these, further expanding treatment options for HIV-positive patients. Combination therapy approaches developed in 1996 were especially effective, and by 1997 a global standard of care had been adopted.

Public policy during this period took a brave step socially. The condom, rarely ever spoken of in polite company and used even less, became less taboo and more widely used than ever before. Condom sales took off in developed countries, quadrupling in some areas. This was due to the efforts of the CDC; similar campaigns in the UK and Europe sought to slow the spread of AIDS by promoting safe sex. President Clinton's administration aggressively advocated for HIV/AIDS education and funneled more federal resources toward AIDS research. Internationally, the WHO AIDS program was replaced by the UNAIDS Global Programme that is still in existence today.

HIV/AIDS in Africa

In most of Africa, public opinion was backed by the leadership of African politicians who refused to acknowledge the existence of sex between men, let alone a health crisis that affected a nation's homosexual population. In many countries, homosexuality was and still is a criminal act; it was not uncommon for early AIDS activists to end up in jail. In countries where the gay social network operated underground, reaching the population with lifesaving education and antiretrovirals was near impossible.

Furthermore, in African nations, public policy was focused on treatment options, versus the needle exchange programs and safe sex awareness campaigns found in other parts of the world. Unfortunately, a lack of trained healthcare professionals made it difficult to administer the medications that might have slowed the rate of HIV infection in these countries.

By 2003, AIDS would overtake swaths of the African continent; nearly 40 percent of Botswana's adult population was infected, with similar percentages in Swaziland. The outlook was especially grim for the children of HIV-positive adults. The US Agency for International Development (USAID) estimated that by 2010, 40 million children in developing African nations would have lost one or both parents to AIDS.

Where We Are Now: 2000 - Today

Since 2000, other factors have begun to contribute to the global spread of HIV. Heroin addiction in Asia has been on the rise, which brought with it dirty needles and the risk of new infections. India suffered with over 2 million diagnoses alone, in spite of the government's refusal to admit the epidemic had adversely affected the nation.

The WHO released its comprehensive report examining HIV and AIDS in all of its 25-year history in 2010. This report had good news for developed nations: by 2008, the US domestic HIV infection rate was considered effectively stable, and has remained so to this day. The report also demonstrated that while insistent public awareness campaigns about safe sex and other methods of transmission had slowed the rate of HIV infection in developed countries. There was much to be done elsewhere.

Global education and aid efforts

In 2003, the WHO announced its "3 by 5 Plan", wherein 3 million people living in undeveloped countries would gain access to treatment by 2005. Financial problems plagued the initiative. Ultimately, private philanthropists and the US government funded the delivery of crucial antiretroviral medication to 15 African countries. The "3 by 5 Plan" was unsuccessful, but it did drive a renewed push by the WHO to deliver care to sub-Saharan Africans by 2010.

HIV denialism disrupts aid

What had begun as a crisis within the medical community had taken on decided political overtones by the mid-2000s. Members of the UN and individual governments operated multiple initiatives; sometimes entire continents were targeted, and sometimes local government strove to reduce infection rates on home turf.

By the time Mbeki was recalled from the presidency in 2008 and one year before the FDA approved its 100th HIV/AIDs drug, an estimated 16.9% of South Africans aged 15 - 49 were HIV positive.

One notable exception to denialism among African national governments was Uganda. Aggressive public awareness efforts educated Ugandans about safe sex and safer drug use, and as a result, the rate of HIV infections was halved over a ten-year period. This success allowed African nations to overcome the societal taboos that prevented frank discussions about safe sex. Globally, public awareness was at its highest since the AIDS crisis had begun, but this awareness had yet to reach sub-Saharan African countries.

virulent [ˈvɪrjʊlənt]	*adj.* of a disease or poison extremely dangerous or harmful and quick to have an effect 致命的；恶性的；剧毒的
strain [streɪn]	*n.* a particular type of plant or animal, or of a disease caused by bacteria, etc. 品系，类型
mortality [mɔːˈtæləti]	*n.* the number of deaths in a particular situation or period of time 死亡率
deprive [dɪˈpraɪv]	*v.* to prevent sb from having or doing sth, especially sth important 剥夺；使丧失；使不能享有
placebo [pləˈsiːbəʊ]	*n.* a substance that has no physical effects, given to patients who do not need medicine but think that they do, or used when testing new drugs（给无实际治疗需要者的）安慰剂；（试验药物用的）无效对照剂
funnel [ˈfʌnəl]	*v.* to send money, information, etc. from various places to someone 使（资金、信息等）汇集，集中
grim [grɪm]	*adj.* unpleasant and depressing 令人不快的；令人沮丧的
overtone [ˈəʊvətəʊn]	*n.* an attitude or an emotion that is suggested and is not expressed in a direct way 弦外之音；言外之意；暗示

2. Q & A on the Regulation on Prevention and Treatment of HIV/AIDS

Read the following passage to complete the note-taking table, and then check your understanding.

Reason of making the Regulation on the Prevention and Treatment of HIV/AIDS ● Prevent and control the occurrence and spread of HIV/AIDS, and ensure (1) _____ _____.

Unit 1 Unit 2 Unit 3 Unit 4 Unit 5 Unit 6 Unit 7 Unit 8

(Continued)

- Build a mechanism of organization and guidance by government with each department (2) _____ respectively.

The authorities that are responsible for this regulation

- The people's governments at or above the county level shall (3) _____, establish and perfect coordinated mechanism and (4) _____ on the work for HIV/AIDS prevention and treatment.
- The competent department of health of the State Council and other relevant departments are in charge of (5) _____ in this work. While the local people's governments at or above the county level are responsible for formulating and (6) _____.
- The state encourages and supports trade unions, communist youth leagues, women's federations, and the Red Cross, and other organizations to assist the people's governments at all levels to (7) _____ for HIV/AIDS prevention and treatment.

The actions that support the work for HIV/AIDS prevention and treatment

- The people's governments at all levels and the relevant departments of the governments shall take measures and make donations for the work of HIV/AIDS prevention, (8) _____ on the group of people with risky behaviors of HIV infection and (9) _____ to the people infected with HIV, AIDS sufferers, and their family members.
- The state encourages and supports the carrying out of scientific research relating to the (10) _____, and treatment of HIV/AIDS, as well as combining (11) _____ and modern medicines.
- The entities and individuals who have made great achievements in and contributions to the work should be gave commendation and awards.
- The local people's governments at all levels and the relevant departments of the governments shall (12) _____ for the publicity of the work.
- The competent departments of health of the people's governments at or above the county level shall strengthen the work for publicity and education, as well as (13) _____ to the relevant departments, organizations and individuals who take part in the publicity.
- Medical institutions shall organize their staff members to (14) _____ on the prevention and treatment of HIV/AIDS.
- The competent departments of education of the people's governments at or above the county level shall guarantee the related knowledge of on HIV/AIDS prevention and treatment can be incorporated into students' education.
- The local people's governments at or above the county level shall (15) _____ for HIV/AIDS prevention and treatment at medical institutions.

Passage C

Q & A on the Regulation on Prevention and Treatment of HIV/AIDS

With the sharp rise of the number of people infected with HIV/AIDS in China in recent years, the issue of prevention and treatment of HIV/AIDS patients has caught the attention of the Chinese government. The governments at all levels in China have put the prevention and treatment of HIV/AIDS on the top of their agenda by formulating laws and regulations to check the spread of the deadly pandemic. Here is a medical student and his teacher discussing the measures taken by the governments to deal with the prevention and treatment of HIV/AIDS throughout China.

Student: Why should we make the Regulation on the Prevention and Treatment of HIV/AIDS?

Teacher: The present Regulation is formulated in accordance with the Law on the Prevention and Treatment of Epidemic Diseases for the purpose of preventing and controlling the occurrence and spread of HIV/AIDS, and ensuring individual and public health.

Student: What are the guidelines for the work of HIV/AIDS prevention and treatment?

Teacher: The guidelines for laying emphasis on prevention, and combining prevention with treatment shall be adhered to for the work of HIV/AIDS prevention and treatment, and the mechanism of organization and guidance by government with each department performing its own functions respectively, and the common participation of the whole society shall be established. Publicity and education shall be strengthened. And such measures as behavioral interventions and care and support shall be adopted to implement comprehensive prevention and treatment.

Student: Should we discriminate against people infected with HIV/AIDS?

Teacher: No entity or individual may discriminate against people infected with HIV/AIDS and their family members. The lawful rights and interests enjoyed by the people infected with HIV/AIDS and their family members in marriage, employment, medical treatment, and education shall be protected by law.

Student: Who will give guidance to the work for prevention and treatment uniformly?

Teacher: The people's governments at or above the county level shall give guidance to the work for prevention and treatment uniformly, establish and perfect coordinated mechanism for the work of HIV/AIDS prevention and treatment and work responsibility system, and make examination and supervision on the work for HIV/AIDS prevention and treatment undertaken by the relevant departments.

The relevant departments of the people's governments at or above the county level shall be responsible for HIV/AIDS prevention and treatment and the supervision and administration thereof according to their divisions of functions.

Student: Who will formulate planning for HIV/AIDS prevention and treatment?

Teacher: The competent department of health of the State Council shall formulate national planning for HIV/AIDS prevention and treatment together with other relevant departments of the State Council. The local people's governments at or above the county level shall, according to the provisions of the present Regulation and the national planning for HIV/AIDS prevention and treatment, formulate and organize the implementation of the action plan for HIV/AIDS prevention and treatment within their own administrative regions.

Student: Who will carry out the work for HIV/AIDS prevention and treatment?

Teacher: The state encourages and supports trade unions, communist youth leagues, women's federations, and the Red Cross, and other organizations to assist the people's governments at all levels to carry out the work for HIV/AIDS prevention and treatment.

The residents' committees and the villagers' committees shall assist the local people's governments at all levels and the relevant departments of the governments to carry out publicity and education on relevant laws, regulations, policies, and knowledge for HIV/AIDS prevention and treatment, develop the public welfare undertakings in respect of HIV/AIDS prevention and treatment, and do a good job for HIV/AIDS prevention and treatment.

Student: What measures shall the people's governments take to encourage and support the relevant organizations and individuals to participate in the work for HIV/AIDS prevention and treatment?

Teacher: The people's governments at all levels and the relevant departments of the governments shall take measures to encourage and support the relevant organizations and individuals to participate in the work for HIV/AIDS prevention and treatment in accordance with the provisions of the present Regulation and the requirements of the national planning for HIV/AIDS prevention and treatment and the action plan for HIV/AIDS prevention and treatment, and make donations on the work for HIV/AIDS prevention and treatment, and conduct behavioral interventions on the group of people with risky behaviors of HIV infection, and provide care and support to the people infected with HIV, AIDS sufferers, and their family members.

Student: Does the state encourage and support the carrying out of scientific research as well as international cooperation and exchange relating to the prevention, diagnosis, and treatment of HIV/AIDS?

Teacher: The state encourages and supports the carrying out of scientific research relating to the prevention, diagnosis, and treatment of HIV/AIDS to improve the scientific and technical level for HIV/AIDS prevention and treatment, encourages and supports the carrying out of clinical treatment and research on HIV/AIDS prevention and treatment through traditional medicines and through combining traditional medicines and modern medicines.

The state encourages and supports the carrying out of international cooperation and exchange on the work for HIV/AIDS prevention and treatment.

Student: Who will be awarded for the work of HIV/AIDS prevention and treatment and who will be given subsidy or preferential treatment of HIV/AIDS?

Teacher: The relevant departments of the people's governments at or above the county level shall give commendation and awards to the entities and individuals who have made great achievements in and contributions to the work for HIV/AIDS prevention and treatment.

Anyone who suffers from AIDS，loses labor capacity，or dies of HIV infection due to his participation in the work for HIV/AIDS prevention and treatment or execution of public affairs shall be given subsidy or preferential treatment of HIV/AIDS.

Student：How shall the local people's governments carry out publicity and education on HIV/AIDS prevention and treatment?

The local people's governments at all levels and the relevant departments of the governments shall set up fixed billboards for HIV/AIDS prevention and treatment or post public welfare advertisements on HIV/AIDS prevention and treatment.

The competent departments of health of the people's governments at or above the county level shall strengthen the work for publicity and education on HIV/ AIDS prevention and treatment，and render technical support to the relevant departments，organizations and individuals that carry out the work for the publicity and education on HIV/AIDS prevention and treatment.

Medical institutions shall organize their staff members to study the relevant laws， regulations，policies，and knowledge on HIV/AIDS prevention and treatment.

The competent departments of education of the people's governments at or above the county level shall give guidance and urge higher education institutions， secondary vocational schools，and regular secondary schools to bring the knowledge on HIV/AIDS prevention and treatment into the relevant curriculum， and carry out the relevant after-school educational activities.

The local people's governments at or above the county level shall open telephone counseling service for HIV/AIDS prevention and treatment at medical institutions，so as to provide the general public with counseling service and guidance for HIV/AIDS prevention and treatment.

adhere [əd'hɪə(r)]	*v*. to stick firmly to sth 黏附；附着
publicity [pʌb'lɪsəti]	*n*. the business of attracting the attention of the public to sth/sb；the things that are done to attract attention 宣传业
discriminate [dɪ'skrɪmɪneɪt]	*v*. to recognize that there is a difference between people or things；to show a difference between people or things 区别；辨别；区分
federation [ˌfedə'reɪʃən]	*n*. a group of clubs，trade/labor unions，etc. that have joined together to form an organization（俱乐部、工会等的）联合会
execution [ˌeksɪ'kjuːʃən]	*n*. the act of doing a piece of work，perform a duty，put a plan into action，etc. 实行；执行；实施

3. **Lexical chunks and sentence rewriting**

A. Substitute the underlined part with the words or expressions you have learned.

(1) If left untreated，HIV can lead to the disease AIDS. (passage A)

Answer:

_____ , HIV can lead to AIDS.

(2) Over time，HIV can destroy so many of these cells that the body can't fight off infections and disease. (passage A)

Answer:

Over time，HIV can destroy so many of these cells that the body can't _____ infections and disease.

(3) Today，a person who is diagnosed with HIV, treated before the disease is far advanced，and stays on treatment can live nearly as long as someone who does not have HIV. (passage A)

Answer:

Today，a person who is diagnosed with HIV and has received treatment and _____ before severe illness _____ those who are not infected with HIV.

(4) Once someone has a dangerous opportunistic illness，life expectancy without treatment falls to about 1 year. (passage A)

Answer:

Once someone has a dangerous opportunistic illness，life expectancy without treatment will _____ about 1 year.

(5) Symptoms are similar to those of the flu and may last anywhere from a few days to several weeks. (passage A)

Answer:

The symptoms are similar to influenza and can _____ .

(6) Treatment helps keep the virus in check. (passage A)

Answer:

Treatment helps _____ .

(7) People who are on ART and stay virally suppressed are much less likely to transmit HIV than those who are not virally suppressed. (passage A)

Answer:

Compared with those who are not inhibited by the virus, _____ and maintain virus suppression are much less likely to transmit HIV.

(8) The first needle exchange programs were instituted; the FDA began to consider whether the nation's supply of banked blood was safe. (Passage B)

Answer:

The first needle exchange programs were _____ ; the FDA began to consider whether the nation's supply of banked blood was safe.

(9) Elsewhere，new cases of AIDS were stacking up in Russia, Ukraine, and other parts of Eastern Europe. (Passage B)

Answer：

Elsewhere，new cases of AIDS were _____ in Russia，Ukraine，and other parts of Eastern Europe.

(10) Meanwhile，research scientists were <u>gaining ground</u> . (Passage B)

Answer：

Meanwhile，research scientists were _____ .

(11) Condom sales <u>took off</u> in developed countries，quadrupling in some areas. (Passage B)

Answer：

Condom sales _____ in developed countries，quadrupling in some areas.

(12) The outlook was especially <u>grim</u> for the children of HIV-positive adults. (Passage B)

Answer：

The outlook was especially _____ for the children of HIV-positive adults.

(13) What had begun as a crisis within the medical community had taken on decided political <u>overtones</u> by the mid-2000s. (Passage B)

Answer：

What had begun as a crisis within the medical community had taken on decided political _____ by the mid-2000s.

B. Rewrite the following sentences using the academic expressions you have learned in the articles.

(1) When the number of your CD4 cells falls below 200 cells per cubic millimeter of blood（200 cells/mm^3），you are considered to have progressed to AIDS.

Lexical chunks： _____

Sentence rewriting： _____

_____

(2) President Clinton's administration aggressively advocated for HIV/AIDS education and funneled more federal resources toward AIDS research.

Lexical chunks： _____

Sentence rewriting： _____

_____

(3) By 2003，AIDS would spread across extensive areas of the African continent.

Lexical chunks： _____

Sentence rewriting： _____

_____

4. **Bilingual translation**

Put the following into Chinese or vice versa.

A. **English-Chinese translation**

Learn the following useful expressions by translating the sentences selected from the passages.

(1) is diagnosed with 被诊断出

Unit 1
Unit 2
Unit 3
Unit 4
Unit 5
Unit 6
Unit 7
Unit 8

Excerpt:

Today, a person who is diagnosed with HIV, treated before the disease is far advanced, and stays on treatment can live nearly as long as someone who does not have HIV.

Translation:

_____

_____

(2) become vulnerable to 容易

Excerpt:

AIDS is the stage of infection that occurs when your immune system is badly damaged and you become vulnerable to opportunistic infections.

Translation:

_____

_____

(3) show symptoms 显示症状

Excerpt:

Some people who have HIV do not show any symptoms at all for 10 years or more.

Translation:

_____

_____

(4) on the grounds 由于……的原因

Excerpt:

Originally a chemotherapy drug, AZT worked so well during its trial that the FDA halted the trial on the grounds that it would be unethical to deprive those patients who received a placebo of the actual drug.

Translation:

_____

_____

(5) take off (产品、活动、事业等)腾飞,突然成功

Excerpt:

Condom sales took off in developed countries, quadrupling in some areas.

Translation:

_____

_____

(6) in spite of 尽管

Excerpt:

Heroin addiction in Asia has been on the rise, which brought with it dirty needles and the risk of new infections. India suffered with over 2 million diagnoses alone, in spite of the government's refusal to admit the epidemic had adversely affected the nation.

Translation:

_____

_____

B. Chinese-English translation

Put the Chinese paragraph into English.

十多年来,她一直致力于与艾滋病和结核病相关的工作,并在多个重大国际活动中呼吁社会各界加大对这两种疾病的关注力度,包括 G20 会议和联合国大会。她在解决艾滋病污名和歧视问题方面所做的努力让更多的人获得了必要的艾滋病诊疗服务。她对儿童和青年人的关注,尤其是那些因艾滋病而成为孤儿的儿童,让更多的人了解了如何帮助儿童艾滋病毒携带者过上有尊严、没有歧视的健康生活。

_____

_____

_____

_____

_____

_____

_____

_____

V. Speaking-out   AIDS Prevention

1. Read and say

There is a group of pictures about AIDS prevention. You can choose one of them and share your understanding of it. Mark down the interesting ideas of your classmates.

Speaking skills:
Read the comics and tell the story. Here are the procedures:
(1) Choose a picture and describe it. Describe what you see, create sentences and inject some new words.
(2) Write down the interesting points and new ideas of your classmates.
(3) Create 10 - 15 sentences relating to the implication of the pictures base on your understanding. Be as creative and imaginative as you can. Attention should be paid to the explicit and implicit meaning of the pictures.
(4) Read the sentences aloud and then start correcting the sentences on your own.
More useful expressions:
HIV sufferers/carriers
passive immunity
prenatal transmission
premarital sex

（Continued）

preconception counseling
prevention education
explosive level
time bomb
downplay the epidemic
high-risk populations
be attributable to
labor mobility
transient population
unprotected sex
autoimmunization
reuse of needles and syringes
to contain the epidemic
in their most sexually active stages of life
heterosexual population
homosexual intercourse
downplay the epidemic
blood-borne diseases

AIDS prevention	Notes

2. Watch and act

Watch a video clip. Fill in the blanks and then act it out in class.

Hello, and welcome to the greatest game show on television — True or False! With your host, Dr. Pill.

Good evening, everybody. Today's subject is HIV. HIV stands for human (1) _____ virus. It is the virus that can lead to the development of the disease AIDS. HIV attacks the body's immune system. Untreated, HIV reduces the number of T cells in the body. T cells are what help your body to (2) _____, and HIV can destroy so many of them that the body becomes (3) _____. Infections and other kinds of illnesses can (4) _____ a very weak immune system.

And now to our contender, Christy! We will give her statements about HIV, and Christy will have to choose whether they are true or false. Are you ready, Christy?

Here is your first statement: You can tell by looking at someone whether they have HIV. You are — correct! The only way to know if a person has HIV is to get an HIV test.

Second statement: You can get HIV through (5) _____, or being near someone with HIV. You are — wrong. Oh — HIV can only be spread through bodily fluids. It can be transmitted through sex, by sharing a drug needle, or being breastfed by someone who has HIV. If a (6) _____ woman is living with HIV and doesn't get the proper treatment before giving birth, her baby could be born with HIV. You cannot get HIV from sharing a glass, (7) _____, or sharing a bathroom with someone who has HIV.

OK, and now for the final round — the quick round! Here is your statement. This product can prevent a person from getting HIV: condoms, birth control pills, a medicine called PrEP. Ah — you are — correct! You got them all right! When you have sex, condoms can help provide protection. And for people (8) _____ for HIV, a doctor can now (9) _____ a medication called PrEP that can be taken to lower their risk.

And we have a winner! Tell her what she won. You win an HIV home testing kit. And from you're back home, remember — once you begin to have sex, it's important that both you and your partner get tested for sexually transmitted diseases and HIV (10) _____. Good night, everybody, and we'll see you next time on True or False!

VI. Pros/Cons HIV and AIDS：Language and the Blame Game

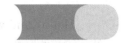

1. Read the following passage with ten statements attached to it. Each statement contains information given in one of the paragraphs. Identify the paragraph from which the information is derived. You may choose a paragraph more than once. Each paragraph is marked with a letter.

_____（1）The reduction of "people/women living with HIV" to a bunch of letters is dehumanizing.

_____（2）"Elimination Plan", a kind of negative language，makes us feel battered and bruised.

_____（3）Too much negative language were heard in International AIDS Society Conference.

_____（4）The potential results of the use of such language should be considered seriously before its application in the global scale.

_____（5）With the language of nature and nurture，we can work together to create a better world.

_____（6）As Lakoff and Johnson have said，language frames the way we think and shapes the world.

_____（7）HIV medication was first introduced in the mid-1990s.

_____（8）Militaristic，combative language is often used in relation to cancer.

_____（9）"Ending gender-based violence" is closely linked to HIV for females.

_____（10）Martha Tholanch thought that mindfulness is vital in the use of language.

A）The negative and dehumanizing language used by scientists discussing global HIV policy is sapping the soul of those on the receiving end. The call for an alternative language of nature and nurture must be heard.

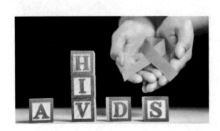

B）While attending the International AIDS Society Conference on Pathogenesis，Treatment and Prevention in Vancouver last week，I posted on my Facebook page："Have retreated from IAS2015 for a breather. Too much negative language about 'loss to follow up'，'defaulters'，'failure to achieve viral suppression'，'shock and kill' strategies against HIV reservoirs is damaging to this soul..."

C）One of many kind responses came from Martha Tholanah："Mindfulness in use of language is important." Am I "lost to follow up" or have I been "bullied out of care"?

D）Global HIV policy is full of dehumanizing, aggressive, militaristic and combative phrases which are deeply depressive，not soothing for the soul. For instance, we people with HIV are often just called "PLHIV" or "WLHIV" short for "people/ women living with HIV." This reduction of an individual to a bunch of letters feels very dehumanizing and I can't think of any other health condition where the individual is so reduced to an acronym. Similarly we are widely said to have been "infected" or to potentially "infect" others. In a word document thesaurus, this translates as "impure, contaminated, perverted, infected..." That doesn't feel great. I have written before on "openDemocracy 50.50" of the euphemism of "Option B+", a strategy that would put pregnant women on lifelong HIV treatment the day they are diagnosed, which is not an option for them — only their governments.

E) Some UN documents, such as the 2013 WHO HIV treatment guidelines, seek for us to "achieve viral suppression" and if we don't, health staff — even some male activists with HIV — brand us as "defaulters", "failures", "wasting resources", and worse, with their targets and goals unmet. Susan Sontag wrote of this "blame the victim" mode long ago and nothing has changed. Even the phrase "lost to follow up" and "treatment-naive patients" also make us sound somehow — well — naive, careless and thoughtless, as if there might not be key intentional reasons for our "failure" to return to a clinic. In a recent trial in South Africa, where it was discovered that young women participants had not in fact made use of a tablet and gel that were being trialed when they said they had, they were deemed by the researchers to have ruined the trial by "lying". As Professor Ida Susser explains: "When a study fails, we must be careful not to imply that the subjects are at fault. My analysis of the study suggests, rather, that the research design was to blame." Other language that depresses includes the ongoing reference to "HIV/ AIDS" as if they are one and the same.

F) Ever since HIV medication was introduced in the mid-1990s, HIV has no longer been a death sentence for those of us privileged enough to access treatment when we need it. Yet this phrase is still used repeatedly by those who should know better.

G) Last week at the Vancouver International AIDS Conference, one plenary presentation on a cure even talked of the virtues of "shock and kill" tactics of using an "aggressive" regime of early treatment to suppress the HIV reservoir which builds up in our bodies after we first acquire HIV. Why do we have to use such combative, militaristic language when we could talk about "reduction" or "management" of the reservoir instead?

H) In response to our frustration over negative language, including that of the "Global Plan Towards the Elimination of New HIV Infections Among Children by 2015 and Keeping Their Mothers Alive", known widely just as the "Elimination Plan", a number of us women living with HIV wrote an article for the *Journal of the International AIDS Society*, to explain why we found such language so debilitating and harmful and to offer alternative, blame-free, woman-positive, language instead. This has slowly gained traction in some corners. But it is yet to be adopted by mainstream HIV scientists, for whom perhaps numbers rather than language are more their comfort zone. Yet, many of us on the receiving end of such language feel battered and bruised by how it saps our souls.

I) The Global Plan above has as its four strategies four "prongs". As I explained in a speech in 2013, prongs remind me of pitch-forks and botched abortions rather than of a global strategy to care and support for women living with HIV as they prepare for motherhood. The potential ramifications of the use of such language should be considered carefully before its use in global policies. Whilst published at global level as voluntary guidelines, it often has dire knock-on effects at the country level. In that speech I also offered an alternative language.

J) Another concept which is curiously negative is the idea of "ending gender-based violence", which is closely connected to HIV for women. In a West African regional workshop in Dakar in 2013, we asked UN staff, government staff and NGO staff alike what kind of world they dream of beyond the end of gender-based violence (GBV). Their common or unified response was "if we have a world without gender-based violence, then we will be out of a job". I found that response immensely revealing about the self-limiting nature of using negative language since they were sub-consciously unable to work towards a world beyond GBV, firstly because such a positive concept had never even been considered and secondly because realizing such a vision would herald their redundancies.

K) Language, as Lakoff and Johnson have explained at length, frames the way we think and shapes our world. If we use negative, combative, problem-focused, competitive, and militaristic language, we think and act accordingly. By contrast, if we use the language of nature, nurture and growth, our thoughts and actions respond creatively — and also turn to positive solutions.

L) Militaristic, combative language is widely used in relation to cancer too — "beating" cancer, "fighting" it and, when someone dies, declaring that she/he has "lost her/his battle with it". But such language, I believe, is both unnecessary and damaging to our souls. I am a great believer in organic gardening, in finding balance in my plot and in not zapping weeds or slugs with toxic chemicals but with living alongside them, accepting them as part of nature's rich tapestry, using physical barriers such as gravel, copper strips and old carpet to contain them instead, so that I can also grow nourishing vegetables safely. If I were to use any spray, I would only use it with extreme caution and in very small quantity. Bugs were here before us and will outlive us. To imagine otherwise is folly indeed.

M) Similarly, I look at my HIV as a part of me which I accept rather than reject. I live alongside it and around it in my body, with modest HIV medication, rather than trying to reject or defeat it. It is not a wholly negative experience. I and many colleagues thank our HIV for giving us many insights into the purpose of our lives and into the injustices which it has brought so many others around the world. I have had many good conversations over the past year with my sister, who has pancreatic cancer. She points out that when people die in the normal course of events, we do not say that they have lost the "battle" to stay alive, but accept it as normal. Though challenged by her cancer, my sister is not fighting it: rather, she is doing all she can to support her immune system so that it can best perform its normal function (cancer has been described as a breakdown of the immune system — the body is hardwired to heal). Recognizing better the impermanence of life, the quality of her life is actually enhanced — this does not sound like "a battle".

N) A more gentle, holistic response to the containment of disease is needed rather than the aggressively-charged metaphors which bombard us all. The one certainty that joins us all as living human beings is our impermanence — that we will die. Atul Gawande and Deepak Chopra have eloquently argued how our attempts to assume otherwise are hubristic and there is often more sense in our seeking to heal rather than to cure ourselves, to find balance in ourselves as our bodies deal with our ailments.

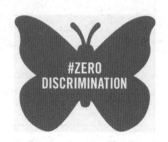

O) The language of nature, nurture, roots, shoots, branches, warmth, rain, growth and creation is something that makes me feel good about myself and others around me. In my garden I need a tool shed, not an arsenal.

P) With our tools, we can join together to create a better world for us all, with greater equity of income, of social, gender and environmental justice, greater involvement in political decision-making in all policies that affect our lives. What will help us along the way is a sense that we have scientists, donors and policymakers working with us, not against us, seeking a shared vision rather than chasing their targets, offering us respect, dignity and appreciation of the trials we face along the way in initiating — and continuing with — our self-care. We all need to work together in this garden and we need to respect the workings of the slugs, bugs and weeds also in our lives.

Q) The forces of nature are bigger than us all and to assume we can overcome them — and to blame people with HIV if we don't — is folly on a grand scale indeed.

2. **Read the following statements. Decide to what extent you agree or disagree with each statement, and write down your own pros or cons in the box, then set out your rational viewpoint and the reasons.**

(1) The negative and dehumanizing language used by scientists discussing global HIV policy is sapping the soul of those on the receiving end.

(2) This reduction of an individual to a bunch of letters feels very dehumanizing.

(3) Language frames the way we think and shapes the world.

(4) A more gentle, holistic response to the containment of disease is needed rather than the aggressively-charged metaphors which bombard us all.

(5) The language of nature, nurture, roots, shoots, branches, warmth, rain, growth and creation is something that makes me feel good about myself and others around me.

Pros	Cons
_____	_____
_____	_____
_____	_____
_____	_____
_____	_____
_____	_____
_____	_____
_____	_____
_____	_____
_____	_____
_____	_____
_____	_____

VII. Outcome Sentence Analysis and Essay Writing

1. **Sentence-structure analysis**

   Analyze the following sentences and draw a tree-structure.

   (1) The global burden of HIV infection in the years to come will be borne overwhelmingly by people in these countries where poverty affects more women than it does men, further increasing their vulnerability to infection.

   (2) If left untreated, HIV reduces the number of CD4 cells (T cells) in the body, making the person more likely to get infections or infection-related cancers.

   (3) People who are taking medicine to treat HIV, and who take their medications right way, every day, may be in this stage for several decades because treatment helps keep the virus in check.

   (4) It's important to remember that people can still transmit HIV to others during this phase even if they have no symptoms, although people who are on ART and stay virally suppressed are much less likely to transmit HIV than those who are not virally suppressed.

(5) Bathhouses and clubs catering to gay clientele were closed down, and law enforcement personnel were issued gloves and masks to protect them against potential exposure.

(6) Originally a chemotherapy drug, AZT worked so well during its trial that the FDA halted the trial on the grounds that it would be unethical to deprive those patients who received a placebo of the actual drug.

2. **Essay writing**

   Write an essay on HIV/AIDS. Search for relevant information via the Internet or books in the library. The following outline is for your reference.

   Outline:

   (1) What is HIV/AIDS?

   (2) How does HIV spread and develop?

   (3) What are the main problems for HIV-infections nowadays?

   (4) What is your advice on HIV prevention or treatment?

Unit **3**
Autism

I. Info-storm Web News on Autism

Read the web page. Then answer the questions orally.

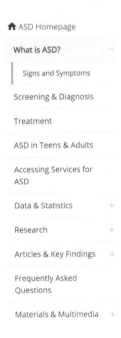

🏠 ASD Homepage

What is ASD?

> Signs and Symptoms

Screening & Diagnosis

Treatment

ASD in Teens & Adults

Accessing Services for ASD

Data & Statistics   +

Research   +

Articles & Key Findings   +

Frequently Asked Questions

Materials & Multimedia   +

What is Autism Spectrum Disorder?

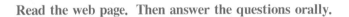

Autism spectrum disorder (ASD) is a <u>developmental disability</u> that can cause significant social, communication and behavioral challenges. There is often nothing about how people with ASD look that sets them apart from other people, but people with ASD may communicate, interact, behave, and learn in ways that are different from most other people. The learning, thinking, and problem-solving abilities of people with ASD can range from gifted to severely challenged. Some people with ASD need a lot of help in their daily lives; others need less.

A diagnosis of ASD now includes several conditions that used to be diagnosed separately: autistic disorder, pervasive developmental disorder not otherwise specified (PDD-NOS), and Asperger syndrome. These conditions are now all called autism spectrum disorder.

Signs and Symptoms

People with ASD often have problems with social, emotional, and communication skills. They might repeat certain behaviors and might not want change in their daily activities. Many people with ASD also have different ways of learning, paying attention, or reacting to things. Signs of ASD begin during early childhood and typically last throughout a person's life.

Children or adults with ASD might:

(1) How can we set people with ASD apart from other people?

_____

(2) What are the treatments available for people with ASD?

_____

(3) What will the people with ASD face during their adolescence and young adulthood?

_____

(4) What services should be provided to people with ASD and their family?

_____

autism spectrum disorder	*n*. conditions commonly manifesting in early childhood and characterized by impaired social or communication skills, repetitive behaviors, or a restricted range of interests 孤独症谱系障碍
interact [ˌɪntərˈækt]	*v*. to communicate with or react to 交流；互相作用
pervasive [pɜːˈveɪsɪv]	*adj*. present or noticeable in every part of a thing or place 充斥各处的；弥漫的，遍布的
Asperger syndrome	a form of autism spectrum disorder that is less severe than other forms, characterized by difficulty with social interaction and communication and by repetitive behavior or restricted interests 阿斯佩格综合征

Unit 1　Unit 2　Unit 3　Unit 4　Unit 5　Unit 6　Unit 7　Unit 8

II. Watching-in　What Is Autism Like?

1. View the video clips. Match the photos (A – D) to the video clips (1 – 4).

A.

B.

GETTING
SOME HELP

C.

COULD MY BUBBA BE
ON THE AUTISM
SPECTRUM?

D.

BUBBAS ON THE
SPECTRUM

Video clip 1：_____　　　　Video clip 2：_____

Video clip 3：_____　　　　Video clip 4：_____

sultana [sʌlˈtɑːnə]	*n.* the dried fruit of a small white seedless grape, originally produced in SW Asia, used in cakes, curries, etc; seedless raisin 无子葡萄干
fussy [ˈfʌsɪ]	*adj.* (of a person) fastidious about one's needs or requirements; hard to please (人)爱挑剔的,难取悦的
texture [ˈtekstʃə(r)]	*n.* the way a surface, substance or piece of cloth feels when you touch it, for example how rough, smooth, hard or soft it is 质地;手感
cuddle [ˈkʌdl]	*v.* to hold sb/sth close in your arms to show love or affection 拥抱;搂抱
muck up	to ruin or spoil; make a mess of 使…一团糟

(1) What makes Ned's story different?

_____

(2) Would changing routines make kids with ASD behave differently?

_____

(3) Why is getting help early so important?

_____

2. **View the video clips again. Fill in the blanks to complete the sentences which can help you get the gist of the content.**

(1)

Meet Ned, he's a five-year-old, lives in a house with his sis Queenie, his mum Liz, his dad Joe and their 1) _____ Flip. Ned loves playing with toy cars. He's a 2) _____ of cheese and sultanas, and his favorite color is green, green pj's, green lunch box, green peas even. Green makes Ned happy. Ned goes to a little school. His teacher Miss Heganty is very tall with long red hair and a booming 3) _____, because kids can sometimes be really

(2)

No two kids on the autism spectrum are the same but there are some 1) _____ behaviors you might pick up on. Sometimes children on the spectrum have trouble talking, playing and being with other people. They might show this by not looking at you, avoiding 2) _____, not smiling or using other 3) _____, talking over the top of you or being really loud when you need them to be quiet. Children on the spectrum sometimes like 4) _____

4) _____ . Some days, Ned spends time in a 5) _____ with another teacher Mrs. Hogan. She's a bit like auntie, but doesn't play with her false teeth. Ned gets to practice his 6) _____ in sounds, jump on the green bean bags and roll green play-dough into balls. Ned loves being with Mrs. Hogan. For the most part, Ned is like the other little ones, but his story is a bit different because Ned has ASD. That 7) _____ autism spectrum disorder, a 8) _____ developmental disorder, which means Ned's the same but different.

and repeating things. They might like to do something over and over and over again, copy words and phrases, saying them repeatedly instead of talking, repeat the same movements like rocking back and forth, keep asking the same question, lining up objects, be 5) _____ eaters only eating certain foods, get upset if routines change, like driving a different way to school. Little ones on the spectrum might have more sensitive 6) _____ like hearing, taste, touch, such as brushing their teeth, which to them feels weird or too much noise, like in a playground or a big family group. Sometimes they might 7) _____ to eat a food because it smells or they don't like the 8) _____ . You might notice these things a little or a lot as early as when they're bubs.

(3)

Bubs on the spectrum under the age of 18 months 1) _____ don't turn when they hear their name called or a voice they know, make eye contact, smile when smiled at, 2) _____ with their eyes, 3) _____ to be picked up, cuddle, 4) _____ Hello or Goodbye, look at you when 5) _____ , make noises to get your attention, want to play with others. If you notice any of these things, it's important to see your doctor or 6) _____ . Getting help early for your bub and family is really important. It means 7) _____ your bub will learn new ways to talk and play and be with people, the better

(4)

Life's better for Ned and his family now. He's been 1) _____ and they're getting some help. His mum and dad, Liz and Joe understand why Ned does things the way he does now and don't get so 2) _____ . Instead of Ned screaming when he's thirsty, he's learning to 3) _____ the fridge to show that he wants a drink. When Liz sees Ned start to 4) _____ his toys or start to rock, she knows something is wrong and can help 5) _____ again. Ned's better at eating his food and using the 6) _____ with a little bit of help. And Grandma and Liz are learning ways to help Ned he or she will do at school and later on in life. You and the family will be able to learn new ways to help bub at home and your bub can go to early 8) _____ where they'll teach him or her how to play and be with other kids. They'll teach your bub ways to get what he or she needs without mucking up.

7) _____ at night. Then everyone gets some sleep. Every day things are slowly getting 8) _____.

III. Leading-in Defining Autism

1. **View a video clip and fill in the blanks. Then define the term "autism" in your own words.**

Autism，Autism Spectrum Disorder，or ASD，is a neurodevelopmental disorder that affects a person's social and communication abilities. Persons with ASD also have areas of (1) _____ and sometimes have (2) _____ behavior and sensory sensitivities. Autism is sometimes associated with strengths in the areas of (3) _____, music，art，math and science. But each person with ASD is (4) _____. Autism is a spectrum disorder and (5) _____ significantly from person to person. Some people with ASD may require significant support in their daily lives，while others may need less support，and some live entirely (6) _____. Changes in brain development associated with autism begin during the (7) _____ period. These changes are associated with differences in genetics. It is possible to diagnose ASD when a child is 18 - 24 months of age. Early behavioral (8) _____ helps children with autism learn to communicate and socially (9) _____, and has a significant impact on long term outcome. Support for learning social and communication skills can be helpful throughout (10) _____ and adulthood.

2. **Read the following passage and answer the questions.**

   (1) What is autism?

   _____

   _____

   (2) Can we judge autistic people by their appearance? Why or why not? How can we tell them from ordinary people?

   _____

   _____

(3) What are the syndromes of autism?

_____

_____

(4) Is autism a disease? What is the possible best treatment?

_____

_____

(5) Why are some people more inclined to suffer autism?

_____

_____

Passage A

An Introduction to Autism

What Is Autism?

When people refer to "autism" today, they are usually talking about Autism Spectrum Disorder (ASD), which is a brain-based disorder characterized by social-communication challenges and restricted repetitive behaviors, activities, and interests.

There is often nothing about how people with ASD look that sets them apart from other people, but people with ASD may communicate, interact, behave, and learn in ways that are different from most other people. The learning, thinking, and problem-solving abilities of people with ASD can range from being gifted to severely challenged. Some people with ASD need a lot of help in their daily lives; others need less.

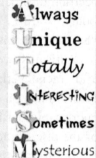

Autism is a spectrum condition. The term "spectrum" reflects the wide variation in challenges and strengths possessed by each person with autism. If you are autistic, you are autistic for life; autism is not an illness or disease and cannot be "cured". Often people feel being autistic is a fundamental aspect of their identity.

How Common Is Autism?

Autism is much more common than most people think. There are around 700,000 people in the UK living with autism — that's more than 1 in 100. People from all nationalities and cultural, religious and social backgrounds can be autistic, although it appears to affect more men than women.

In 2016, the Centres for Disease Control's Autism and Developmental Disabilities Monitoring (ADDM) reported that approximately 1 in 68 children in the United States has been identified with ASD. This rate remains the same as in 2014, which is the first time it has not risen. However, with respect to older data, this new estimate is roughly 30 percent higher than the previous estimate of 1 in 88 children reported in 2012. In the 1980s, autism prevalence was reported as 1 in 10,000. In the nineties, prevalence was 1 in 2,500 and later 1 in 1,000.

What Causes Autism?

Scientists are unsure what, if any, environmental triggers may be involved in autism. One theory, popular in the late 1990s and early 2000s, that vaccines cause autism, has since been disproven by numerous studies conducted around the world.

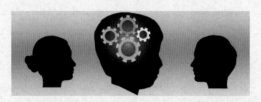

There is no known single cause for autism, although the best available science points to important genetic components. Through twin studies, scientists have determined that autism is a genetically based condition. If one identical (monozygotic) twin has autism, then there is an 36%–95% chance that the other twin will also be diagnosed with an autism spectrum disorder. For non-identical (dizygotic) twins the chance is about 0–31% that both twins will develop autism spectrum disorder. The chance that siblings will both be affected by ASD is also about 2%–18%.

Who Are More Likely to Be Affected by Autism?

Autism is two to five times more likely to affect boys than girls, and is found in all racial, ethnic, and social groups. Until recently, brain experts haven't focused much on the possible gender-based reasons for this difference. Now, in a report published in *JAMA Psychiatry*, scientists point to one possible explanation for the discrepancy.

Brain scientists know that some structures in the brain differ between the sexes. One is the thickness of the cortex, the brain's outer layer that is embedded with nerves involved in memory, thinking, language and other higher cognitive functions. Men tend to have thinner cortex measurements, while women tend to have thicker ones, and this difference is a pretty reliable way to distinguish males from females.

"The assumption was that if the male brain were more vulnerable to ASD, then maybe the brains of females with autism have features that resemble the more male-like brain," says Ecker, a professor of neuroscience and brain imaging at Goethe University in Germany.

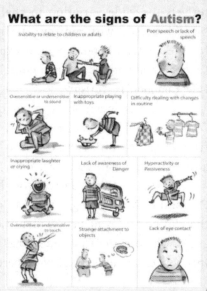

What Are the Signs of Autism?

Every child is different and every child develops at his or her own pace. However, there are specific developmental milestones that all children should be reaching by specific ages.

Possible signs of autism in babies and toddlers:

- By 6 months, no social smiles or other warm, joyful expressions directed at people
- By 6 months, limited or no eye contact
- By 9 months, no sharing of vocal sounds, smiles or other nonverbal communication
- By 12 months, no babbling
- By 12 months, no use of gestures to communicate (e.g. pointing, reaching, waving, etc.)
- By 12 months, no response to name when called
- By 16 months, no words
- By 24 months, no meaningful, two-word phrases
- Any loss of any previously acquired speech, babbling or social skills

Possible signs of autism at any age:

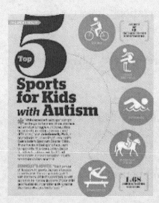

- Avoids eye contact and prefers to be alone.
- Struggles with understanding other people's feelings.
- Remains nonverbal or has delayed language development.
- Repeats words or phrases over and over (echolalia).
- Gets upset by minor changes in routine or surroundings.
- Has highly restricted interests.
- Performs repetitive behaviors such as flapping, rocking or spinning.
- Has unusual and often intense reactions to sounds, smells, tastes, textures, lights and/or colors.

How Do Physicians Screen and Diagnose Autism?

If you've been noticing some early signs of autism in your child, and have brought your concerns to a physician, the next step will be a visit to a physician. Diagnosing ASD can be difficult, since there is no medical test, like a blood test, to diagnose the disorders. Doctors will conduct diagnostic assessments on your child, looking at the child's behavior and development.

ASD can sometimes be detected at 18 months or younger. By age 2, a diagnosis by an experienced professional can be considered very reliable. However, many children do not receive a final diagnosis until much older. This delay means that children with an ASD might not get the help they need.

What Is the Possible Effective Treatment for Autism?

Scientists agree that the earlier in life a child receives early intervention services the better the child's prognosis. All children with autism can benefit from early intervention, and some may gain enough skills to be able to attend mainstream school.

The most effective treatments available today are applied behavioral analysis （ABA）, occupational therapy, speech therapy, physical therapy, and pharmacological therapy. Treatment works to minimize the impact of the core features and associated deficits of ASD and to maximize functional independence and quality of life.

ABA works to systematically change behavior based on principles of learning derived from behavioral psychology. It encourages positive behaviors and discourages negative behaviors. In addition, it teaches new skills and applies those skills to new situations.

variation [ˌveərɪˈeɪʃən]	*n.* the act, process, or accident of varying in condition, character, or degree 变化，变异
prevalence [ˈprevələns]	*n.* the condition of being prevalent, or widespread（疾病等的）流行程度
vaccine [ˈvæksiːn]	*n.* a substance which contains a weak form of the bacteria or virus that causes a disease and is used to protect people from that disease 疫苗
component [kəmˈpəʊnənt]	*n.* a constituent part; element; ingredient 组成部分；成分
monozygotic [ˌmɒnəʊzaɪˈgɒtɪk] **twin**	developed from a single fertilized ovum, as identical twins 同卵双胞胎
dizygotic [ˌdaɪzaɪˈgɒtɪk] **twin**	（of twins） developed from two separately fertilized eggs 异卵双胞胎
affect [əˈfekt]	*v.*（of pain, disease, etc.）to attack or lay hold of sb（疾病）侵袭
JAMA	Journal of the American Medical Association 美国医学协会杂志
outer layer	外层（细胞次生壁外面的一层）
cognitive [ˈkɒgnɪtɪv]	*adj.* of, characterized by, involving, or relating to cognition 认知的

neuroscience [ˌnjʊərəʊˈsaɪəns]	*n*. the field of study encompassing the various scientific disciplines dealing with the structure, development, function, chemistry, pharmacology, and pathology of the nervous system 神经科学
echolalia [ˌekəʊˈleɪlɪə]	*n*. the act of repeating everything sb says, as a result of a mental condition 模仿言语,言语模仿症
flap [flæp]	*v*. to move (wings, arms, etc.) up and down 挥动,舞动(手臂)
spin [spɪn]	*v*. to turn round and round quickly 快速旋转
assessment [əˈsesmənt]	*n*. judging or forming an opinion about sb/sth 评估;评定;鉴定
deficit [ˈdefɪsɪt]	*n*. a deficiency or impairment in mental or physical functioning 身心缺陷;身心功能方面的不健全

3. **Match each of the terms listed below with the numbered definition. Write the letter in the space provided.**

A. trigger	B. embed	C. physician
D. discrepancy	E. repetitive	F. prognosis
G. vulnerable	H. cortex	I. nonverbal
J. pharmacology	K. psychiatry	L. reliable

(1) _____ : to cause to be an integral part of a surrounding whole
(2) _____ : the outer layer of an internal organ or body structure
(3) _____ : a prediction of the probable course and outcome of a disease
(4) _____ : the branch of medicine that deals with the diagnosis, treatment, and prevention of mental and emotional disorders
(5) _____ : divergence or disagreement, as between facts or claims; difference
(6) _____ : something that precipitates a particular event or situation
(7) _____ : capable of being relied on; dependable
(8) _____ : the science of drugs, including their composition, uses, and effects
(9) _____ : a person trained and licensed to practice medicine; one who has a Doctor of Medicine or a Doctor of Osteopathic Medicine degree
(10) _____ : given to or characterized by repetition
(11) _____ : susceptible to physical harm or damage
(12) _____ : involving little or no use of words

IV. Critical Reading　Further Reading on Autism

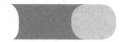

1. A News Report About Autistics

Read the following passage and complete the exercises that follow.

A. Fill in the blanks to complete the table.

Cai's story	● Cai was first diagnosed with ASD at (1)_____ years old. ● Although Cai attended a special needs kindergarten，he finished his nine-year (2) _____ in an inclusive environment in public schools. ● The training program has allowed Cai and 14 other students with special needs to further their studies by attending Shanghai Nanhu (3) _____.
Government measures	● Shanghai has introduced a string of policies to promote (4) _____ for people with mental disorders over the past decade. ● Chinese authorities offer (5) _____ to companies that hire people certified as disabled.
Facts	● Employers remain highly (6) _____ to hire people with autism. ● A report published in 2014 suggested that (7) _____ of people with autism are employed. ● Companies sometimes hire disabled workers on (8) _____ simply to qualify for a tax cut.
Expectations of autistic people's parents	● Cai will be able to (9) _____ when parents get too old or pass away. ● For years, Cai's mother has done everything she can to help Cai become as (10) _____ as possible. ● Autistic people will be provided with a better chance of securing (11) _____ paid work.

B. Judge whether the following statements are true (T) or false (F).

_____ (1) Cai's family members are all excited about his graduation.

_____ (2) The overwhelming majority of autistic children never finish higher education.

_____ (3) Some families with autistic children haven't applied for a disability certificate，as they disagree with classifying their children as "disabled" and worry the label will lead to social stigma.

_____ (4) Most companies show sympathy to the kids with autism and offer them some jobs.

_____ (5) Cai's mother believes work would provide Cai with the regular social interaction and responsibility that he needs.

Passage B

A News Report about Autistics

SHANGHAI — Cai Lechen has been beating the odds since he was first diagnosed with autism spectrum disorder at 2 years old.

The vast majority of children with autism never finish junior high school, let alone go on to higher education. But in 2017 Cai did exactly that, winning a spot on a new government-sponsored training program for students with special needs, which admitted just 15 people that year.

Cai enrolled in hotel management at a Shanghai vocational school, and for the next three years diligently mastered the arts of tea ceremonies, towel origami, and tidying rooms to five-star standards. Now aged 19, he's finally about to complete his degree.

Yet as Cai's graduation day approaches, his family's mood isn't one of celebration, but of foreboding.

"With kids like ours, families look forward to the day when they grow up," Mei Li, Cai's mother, tells Sixth Tone at her home in central Shanghai. "But at the same time, we're afraid of it."

Though bursting with pride at her son's achievements, Mei knows they may count for little when Cai enters the harsh world of job market. Despite efforts to promote inclusivity over recent years, employers remain highly reluctant to hire people with autism.

"We don't know how he'll be able to support himself when we get too old or pass away," Mei tells Sixth Tone. "Most of the autistic kids we know just return home after they finish school or are forced to leave school."

There are an estimated 14 million people with autism spectrum disorder, but only a fraction of this group are in paid work. A report published in 2014 suggested that fewer than 10% of people with autism are employed.

This report, moreover, was based on a survey of around 3,000 families selected by schools, nonprofits, and other organizations supporting those with autism, which are more likely to be actively searching for jobs for their children. Experts tell Sixth Tone the real employment rate is likely far lower.

"There are extremely limited employment opportunities for autistic adults," says Zhou Jinlian, director of Rongaixing, a Guangzhou-based nonprofit that promotes inclusive education for children with autism.

According to Zhou, most companies are highly profit-driven and unwilling to make the extra investment necessary to train and supervise an autistic member of staff.

In southern city Guangzhou, the only companies that hire employees with autism are a handful of large firms that do so as part of their corporate social responsibility strategies, Zhou says. In most cases, these "public welfare posts" don't last long.

"For companies, eventually they need to make money," says Zhou. "Given the not-so-optimistic economic situation, they're even less willing to give autistic applicants a try."

For years, Mei has done everything she can to help Cai become as socially integrated as possible. Aside from his studies, Cai plays badminton every week and is about to sit his grade eight piano test. He tends to speak in short sentences, but he can communicate clearly.

When Sixth Tone asks Cai about what he wants to do after graduation, Mei whispers in his ear: "I want to become a useful person," which he dutifully repeats.

Before several years, Mei's family was hopeful that Cai might one day be able to find work. Shanghai has introduced a string of policies to promote inclusivity for people with mental disorders over the past decade, and things appeared to be improving gradually.

"My son has been very lucky," says Mei. "Although he attended a special needs kindergarten, he finished his nine-year compulsory education in an inclusive environment in public schools. We didn't dare imagine he could further his studies by attending vocational school. But it was made possible with the local government's progressive policies."

The training program, launched by the central Hongkou District in 2017, has allowed Cai and 14 other students with special needs to attend Shanghai Nanhu Vocational School, where they have been learning the skills required to work in the hospitality sector.

"I like folding tablecloths, doing tea ceremonies, and putting things in order the most," Cai tells Sixth Tone.

As part of the program, the students were supposed to intern at the Broadway Mansions Hotel — the iconic, five-star hotel overlooking Shanghai's Bund — this year. The school, however, cancelled all its internship plans after suspending classes in the wake of flu.

For Mei, it's a shame Cai missed out on the opportunity. But ultimately, the internships are of little use anyway, unless they provide students with a better chance of securing permanent, paid work. At the moment, that often isn't the case, she suggests.

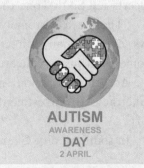

"Every year on April 2 (World Autism Awareness Day) ... companies come to events to demonstrate their corporate social responsibility," says Mei. "But instead of such displays, we need real jobs provided for kids like my son."

Broadway Mansions Hotel has never hired a staff member with a mental disorder before, the hotel's human resources manager, surnamed Li, confirmed to Sixth Tone during a phone call. "We're above all a hotel that requires staff to communicate with our guests. We're not a factory," says Li. "Sympathizing with the kids and their families is one thing, but offering them jobs is another."

Li added that Nanhu Vocational School had invited her to observe its classes for special needs students in the past. "There are possibilities for us to hire one or two of these graduates, but we're not obliged to do so," she says.

While Mei says she understands that companies need to make a profit, she wishes more could be done to help families like hers. Chinese authorities offer tax incentives to companies that hire people certified as disabled, but the impact of this policy has been limited.

Over 20% of families with autistic children haven't applied for a disability certificate, according to the 2014 report, as they disagree with classifying their children as "disabled" and worry the label will lead to social stigma. In practice, moreover, companies sometimes hire disabled workers on low-wage contracts simply to qualify for a tax cut, Mei says. The firms won't even allow their newly hired staff members to attend work, fearing they'll be disruptive, she adds.

"They'll still pay the staff their salaries, but that's not what my family wants," says Mei.

Beyond the issue of financial security, work would provide Cai with the regular social interaction and responsibility that he needs, Mei believes. She can't bear the idea of her son simply staying in the house all day long, as do so many others with his disorder.

"We have to keep him in a social environment to force him to open up," Mei says. "We've been making efforts on this path for over 10 years. If the eventual outcome is our son coming back home, that's unacceptable for us."

The mother even says she'd be willing to quit her own job to support Cai in the workplace full time, or allow Cai to work for free.

"Even if they don't give him a penny in income, we don't mind," says Mei. "We just want him to remain part of wider society."

origami [ˌɒrɪˈɡɑːmɪ]	*n.* the art of making objects for decoration by folding sheets of paper into shapes 折纸艺术
foreboding [fɔːˈbəʊdɪŋ]	*n.* a feeling that sth very bad is going to happen soon 不祥的预感
inclusivity [ˌɪnkluːˈsɪvɪtɪ]	*n.* the quality of trying to include many different types of people and treat them all fairly and equally 包容性

intern [ɪnˈtɜːn]	*v.* to work for a short time in order to obtain practical experience of a type of work 实习
incentive [ɪnˈsentɪv]	*n.* sth that encourages a person to work harder, start a new activity, etc. 激励;刺激
stigma [ˈstɪɡmə]	*n.* a strong feeling of disapproval that most people in a society have about sth, especially when this is unfair 污名;耻辱
disruptive [dɪsˈrʌptɪv]	*adj.* tending to damage the orderly control of a situation 分裂的;破坏性的

2. Traditional Chinese Medicine and Autism

Read the following passage to complete the note-taking table, and then check your understanding.

Classification as in TCM	The "delays" are observed in the areas of (1)_____, (2)_____, (3)_____, (4)_____ and (5)_____. This type of brain dysfunction in children, classic autism characteristic, is seen in traditional Chinese medicine as an imbalance of body functions. Based in the *yin/yang* theory, TCM views disease within the framework of energy balance.
The core of TCM	Chinese medicine sees the (6)_____ as part of the same circular system with the (7)_____. Western medicine has traditionally considered emotional influence on the organs as secondary, while Chinese medicine has always seen it as a key to understanding and achieving balance.
Effect brought by autism in TCM: the heart	In Chinese medicine, (8)_____, which are strongly affected by autism, are primarily ruled by three organ systems: the heart, spleen and kidney. The heart holds the mind or *shen* and rules the mental functions, including the emotional state of the individual and short-term memory.
The spleen	The spleen is linked to the mind's ability to (9)_____.
The kidney *qi*	Kidney *qi* rules over (10)_____. A disturbance in these areas can lead to displays of any autism characteristic.

Passage C

Traditional Chinese Medicine and Autism

According to the National Institute of Child Health and Human Development, current estimated cases of autism range from one in every 1,000 to one in every 500. Theories suggest vaccines are responsible, but there is growing concern that environmental toxins and pollution may be contributing factors. It is also theorized that nutrition, viral infections, immunizations, and antibiotics may be causal aspects as well.

People speak in terms of children "developing" autism, but new research cited by the Autism Society of America suggest genetic ties — that the disorder is present prenatal. An autism symptom will usually appear before the age of three, at which age a formal diagnosis can be made. Because an autism characteristic can be any combination of insufficiencies in language, social communication, and cognition, autism is difficult to diagnose before normal development in these areas would usually occur.

Autism is considered a spectrum disorder by standard medicine. Spectrum disorders are defined as a group of conditions that have similar features but may present an autism symptom in different ways. Autism spectrum disorder (ASD) includes "classic" autism, Asperger syndrome, Rett syndrome, and Pervasive Developmental Disorder Not Otherwise Specified (atypical autism). Each of these conditions usually is accompanied by a secondary autism characteristic such as aggression, irritability, stereotypes (involuntary but seemingly purposeful movement), hyperactivity, negativism, volatile emotions, temper tantrums, short attention span, and obsessive-compulsive behavior.

Autism in the Western medical sense does not exist in Chinese medicine. Instead, it is classified under the Syndrome of 5 Delays. The "delays" are observed in the areas of standing, walking, hair growth, teeth eruption and speech. This type of brain dysfunction in children, classic autism characteristic, is seen in traditional Chinese medicine as an imbalance of body functions. Based in the *yin/yang* theory, TCM views disease within the framework of energy balance.

Unlike Western medicine, which rates the brain the most important factor of the human physique, Chinese medicine sees the body and mind as part of the same circular system with the organs and the central nervous system. Western medicine has traditionally considered emotional influence on the organs as secondary, while Chinese medicine has always seen it as a key to understanding and achieving balance.

In Chinese medicine, reason and awareness, which are strongly affected by autism, are primarily ruled by three organ systems: the heart, spleen and kidney. The heart holds the mind or *shen* and rules the mental functions, including the emotional state of the individual and short-term memory. The spleen is linked to the mind's ability to study, memorize, and concentrate. Kidney *qi* rules over long-term memory. A disturbance in these areas can lead to displays of any autism characteristic.

According to Mary Cissy Majebe's "Chinese Medicine and Autism: An Introduction for Parents, Teachers and Allopathic Physicians", autism treatment includes eliminating phlegm; tonifying heart blood, *qi* and *yin*; clearing heart heat; and tonifying spleen *qi* and kidney essence.

Eliminating phlegm is crucial because it is involved with the two primary Chinese medicine diagnoses of autism. Phlegm misting the mind leads to dull wit and incoherent speech, mental confusion, lethargy and limited attention to surroundings. The condition of phlegm fire harassing the heart presents as disturbed sleep, talking to oneself, uncontrolled laughing or crying, short temper and tendency toward constipation and aggression.

Balance in the heart is another key element because heart blood or *yin* deficiency, as well as heart fire will prompt an autism symptom on different extremes such as lethargy and quietness, fidgety restlessness, or aggressive behaviors.

Spleen *qi* deficiency and kidney essence deficiency are central to the pathology of autism, the former affecting food intake (no interest in food, or an excessive hunger), while the latter will result in poor mental development.

The Autism Research Institute asserts that nutritional treatments have shown great success in autism treatment. They suggest for an autism diet avoiding yeast, glutens, casein, and any allergens. The Chinese medical diet is determined by flavor (pungent, sweet, salty), temperature (both physical and energy quality) and action on the body. Central to the philosophy and practice of Chinese medicine, it is thought that many, if not most, of our health problems are related to imbalances in our diet. Sensitivity to foods is not the cause of autism, but it does appear that certain components of foods exacerbate some of autism's symptoms. Dietary therapy, by creating a healthy autism diet, helps patients treat illness and maintain health. The general rule in Chinese diet therapy is, "Warm foods restore balance. Just go to the center and forget either extreme."

Autism has also been treated with acupuncture and massage. These two methods can be a difficult undertaking. It can take time for a child to adjust to touch treatments, but the benefits that have been discovered through studies and by practitioners may well be worth any required patience.

Acupuncture has made incredible strides in treating autism. Its efficacy can possibly be explained through the medical theory that autism is in part a neuroendocrine dysfunction and a result of the incorrect production of opioids. According to the book *Scientific Bases of Acupuncture*, acupuncture affects opioids, the central nervous system and neuroendocrine function.

Tongue acupuncture is also showing remarkable headway healing dysfunctions related to autism, according to recent studies. It is being studied for treating a number of brain disorders in children, including blindness, cerebral palsy and autism.

Tongue diagnosis is a central piece of the Chinese medical diagnostic system because the tongue is the only organ that can be seen externally. Its condition — color, thickness, dryness, smell and superficial growth reflects the condition of the heart and helps doctors determine treatment.

Although alternative autism treatment such as tongue acupuncture and dietary changes should still be viewed as a complementary approach，these exciting early findings stand as an innovative starting point for a new system of autism treatment.

prenatal [ˌpriːˈneɪtəl]	*adj*. relating to unborn babies and the care of pregnant women 产前的
irritability [ˌɪrɪtəˈbɪlətɪ]	*n*. quick excitability to annoyance 易怒；烦躁
hyperactivity [ˌhaɪpərǽkˈtɪvətɪ]	*n*. a condition characterized by excessive restlessness and movement 极度活跃；活动过度
volatile [ˈvɒlətaɪl]	*adj*. changing easily from one mood to another 易变的；无定性的；无常性的
tantrum [ˈtæntrəm]	*n*. a sudden short period of angry, unreasonable behaviour, especially in a child（尤指儿童）耍脾气，使性子
span [spæn]	*n*. the length of time that sth lasts or is able to continue 持续时间
phlegm [flem]	*n*. the thick substance that forms in the nose and throat, especially when you have a cold 痰
tonify [ˈtəʊnɪfaɪ]	*v*. to make a part of the body firmer, smoother and stronger，by exercise or by applying special creams, etc.（通过锻炼或涂特殊的护肤霜等）改善（身体部位）状况
spleen [spliːn]	*adj*. a small organ near the stomach that controls the quality of the blood cells 脾
lethargy [ˈleθədʒɪ]	*n*. the state of not having any energy or enthusiasm for doing things 无精打采；没有热情；冷漠
restlessness [ˈrestlɪsnɪs]	*n*. an uneasy or nervous state 焦躁不安
efficacy [ˈefɪkəsɪ]	*n*. capacity or power to produce a desired effect 功效，效力

Unit 1 Unit 2 Unit 3 Unit 4 Unit 5 Unit 6 Unit 7 Unit 8

3. **Lexical chunks and sentence rewriting**

   A. **Substitute the underlined part with the words or expressions you have learned.**

   （1）People from all nationalities and cultural，religious and social backgrounds <u>can be autistic</u>，although it appears to affect more men than women.（Passage A）

Answer：

People from all nationalities and cultural，religious and social backgrounds _____ ，although autism seems to affect more men than women.

(2) Scientists are unsure what，if any，<u>environmental triggers may be involved in autism</u>. (Passage A)

Answer：

Scientists are not sure what，if any，_____ .

(3) Mei has done everything she can to <u>help Cai become as socially integrated as possible</u>. (Passage B)

Answer：

Mei has done her best to _____ .

(4) The school，however，cancelled all its internship plans <u>after</u> suspending classes <u>in the wake of</u> flu. (Passage B)

Answer：

However，_____ the outbreak of flu，the school suspended classes _____ cancelled all internship plans.

(5) For Mei，it's a <u>shame</u> Cai <u>missed out on the opportunity</u>. (Passage B)

Answer：

For Mei，it's a _____ that Cai _____ .

(6) But ultimately，the internships <u>are of little use anyway</u>，unless they provide students with a better chance of <u>securing</u> permanent，paid work. (Passage B)

Answer：

But ultimately，the internships _____ unless they provide students with better chance of _____ permanent and paid jobs.

(7) People speak in terms of children "developing" autism，but new research <u>cited</u> by the Autism Society of America suggest genetic ties — that the disorder is present prenatal. (Passage C)

Answer：

People speak in terms of children "developing" autism，but new research _____ by the Autism Society of America suggest genetic ties — that the disorder is present prenatal.

(8) Balance in the heart is another key element because heart blood or *yin* deficiency，as well as heart fire will <u>prompt</u> an autism symptom on different extremes such as lethargy and quietness，fidgety restlessness，or aggressive behaviors. (Passage C)

Answer：

Balance in the heart is another key element because heart blood or *yin* deficiency，as well as heart fire will _____ an autism symptom on different extremes such as lethargy and quietness，fidgety restlessness，or aggressive behaviors.

(9) It does appear that certain <u>components</u> of foods exacerbate some of autism's symptoms. (Passage C)

Answer:

It does appear that certain _____ of foods exacerbate some of autism's symptoms.

B. Rewrite the following sentences using the academic expressions you have learned in the articles.

(1) The most effective treatments available today are applied behavioral analysis (ABA), occupational therapy, speech therapy, physical therapy, and pharmacological therapy. (Passage A)

Lexical chunks: _____

Sentence rewriting: _____

_____

(2) Shanghai has introduced a string of policies to promote inclusivity for people with mental disorders over the past decade, and things appeared to be improving gradually. (Passage B)

Lexical chunks: _____

Sentence rewriting: _____

_____

(3) Sympathizing with the kids and their families is one thing, but offering them jobs is another. (Passage B)

Lexical chunks: _____

Sentence rewriting: _____

_____

(4) Beyond the issue of financial security, work would provide Cai with the regular social interaction and responsibility that he needs. (Passage B)

Lexical chunks: _____

Sentence rewriting: _____

_____

(5) Theories suggest vaccines are responsible, but there is growing concern that environmental toxins and pollution may be contributing factors. (Passage C)

Lexical chunks: _____

Sentence rewriting: _____

_____

4. **Bilingual translation**

Put the following into Chinese or vice versa.

A. **English-Chinese translation**

Learn the following useful expressions by translating the sentences selected from the passages.

(1) Until recently, sb hasn't done sth 某人直到最近还没有……

Excerpt:

Until recently, brain experts haven't focused much on the possible gender-based reasons for this difference.

Translation：

_____

_____

（2）there is a ... chance 有······的可能性

Excerpt：

If one identical（monozygotic）twin has autism then there is a 36%－95% chance that the other twin will also be diagnosed with an autism spectrum disorder.

Translation：

_____

_____

（3）beat the odds 战胜；挑战；由劣势取胜

Excerpt：

He has been beating the odds since he was first diagnosed with autism spectrum disorder at 2 years old.

Translation：

_____

_____

（4）burst with pride 充满自豪　　count for little 无足轻重；算不了什么

Excerpt：

Though bursting with pride at her son's achievements，Mei knows they may count for little when Cai enters the harsh world of job market.

Translation：

_____

_____

（5）... is one thing, ... is another ······是一回事，······又是另一回事

Excerpt：

Sympathizing with the kids and their families is one thing，but offering them jobs is another.

Translation：

_____

_____

B. Chinese-English translation

Put the Chinese paragraph into English.

一年一度的"世界提高孤独症意识日"鼓励人们了解孤独症患者及其亲属所遭受的不可接受的歧视、虐待与孤立，并提升关注与采取行动。正如《残疾人权利公约》所强调的，孤独症患者与常人拥有相等的法律地位，享有同等的人权和基本权利。每年的活动日都会围绕一个主题展开，例如"为全纳教育打开大门"，或正如我们的项目简介所言："就业——孤独症的优势"。

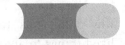

V. Speaking-out Functional Levels of Autism

1. Read and say

Look at the picture describing the three functional levels of autism. Work in pairs and describe the average traits and needed assistance to your partner.

Three Functional Levels of Autism

written from an autistic perspective

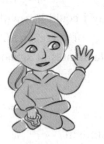
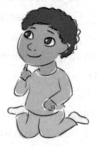
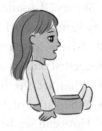

Level 1	Level 2	Level 3
Requiring Support	**Requiring Substantial Support**	**Requiring Very Substantial Support**
I need help navigating a non-autistic world.	*I need help handling everyday challenges.*	*I often need one-on-one support.*
Average traits	**Average traits**	**Average traits**
People may see me as awkward, not disabled.	People can usually tell that I have a disability.	My disability is very obvious.
I can befriend or date non-disabled people, but it's hard and I'm often lonely.	My social life is very limited or nonexistent.	I usually only communicate to express needs or answer questions.
I can handle change, but I prefer routine.	Coping with change is very challenging.	Change and transitions can be unbearably difficult.
My fidgeting is seen as quirky or "annoying."	My repetitive behaviors are noticeably unusual.	My intense repetitive behavior is calming and important to me.
People may think my developmental delays are signs of laziness or insecurity.	I have significant developmental delays and will meet milestones late.	I have large developmental delays and may not meet every milestone.
Please know that	**Please know that**	**Please know that**
Social interactions are challenging. Please be understanding and offer help.	I may seem inattentive, but I hear and understand you.	I may seem unresponsive, but I hear and understand you.
I struggle more than I let on.	Routines and repetitive behavior help me feel safe.	Routines and repetitive behaviors help me feel safe.
Meeting others' expectations is exhausting. Please be patient.	I need a lot of help coping with stress.	I need help with communication skills.
I deserve respect and support.	I deserve respect and support.	I deserve respect and support.

These levels aren't clear-cut or permanent. Someone's skills may change.
Stress, environment, and support will impact someone's ability to function.

2. Watch and act

A. Watch a video clip and fill in the blanks.

Narrator 1：This is the story of a boy who didn't talk for a long time. The boy liked things to always be (1) _____. Any changes would （2） _____ him. The unknown was an （3） _____ place. The boy was very （4） _____ to lights and sounds. So he built （5） _____ hiding

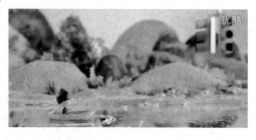

places where they couldn't get in. The boy didn't like looking people in the eye. He wasn't trying to be (6) _____. It just made him feel (7) _____. Sometimes，he'd flap his arms again and again.

Jacob：One day I found out I had something called (8) _____. My family got me help. Slowly，I found my (9) _____ and learned all the way I could live with it better.

Narrator 2：Early intervention can make a (10) _____ of difference.

B. Give a speech on how we can help the bullied autistic classmates at school.

Suggested outline of the speech：

- What are the traits of autism?
- What kind of bullying are faced by autistic students?
- How can we help the bullied autistic classmates as a student?

Speaking skills：give advice in English

- **Use a modal verb：should，ought to**

There are two modal verbs we often use for giving advice："should" and "ought to". Both mean the same thing but work in slightly different ways. Let's look at some examples.

> You should do more travelling.
>
> You shouldn't drink so much beer.

As you can see above，after "should" we use an infinitive without "to".

> You ought to do more travelling.
>
> You ought not to drink so much beer.

- **Make it into a question："Why don't you . . . ?"and "How about . . . ?"**

To make advice less direct，we can use a question to make the person we are advising consider about the advice we are giving them.

> Why don't you do some more tidying?
>
> How about doing some more tidying?

With the question "Why don't you . . ."，we use an infinitive without "to". When we use "How about . . ." to make a question，we use a gerund after it.

- **Put yourself in the person's position："If I were you，I would . . ."**

If someone is asking for your advice，sometimes it's useful to imagine yourself being in that person's position. This is a good way to explain your advice，too.

If I were you, I would travel more.

Remember to use an infinitive after "would" and not "to". To make this negative, put "not" after "would".

- **Use the words "suggest" or "recommend"**

A suggestion or recommendation is another good way of giving advice that isn't too direct. You can use the words "suggest" or "recommend" as in the example below.

I would suggest doing more of an effort.

I would recommend doing this instead.

Use "verb + ing" after "suggest" or "recommend" to explain your advice to the listener. To make these negative, put "not" before your "verb+ing".

- **Advise in a stronger way: "You had better ..."**

Sometimes, you need to make your advice stronger to let the listener know that it's really important. We can use the expression "you had better ..." to do this.

You had (You'd) better start working on your homework.

You had (You'd) better finish this assignment in time.

We use an infinitive after "better" to explain our advice and add "not" after "better" to make the sentence negative.

VI. Pros/Cons Celebrities with Autism

1. **Read the following passage with ten statements attached to it. Each statement contains information given in one of the paragraphs. Identify the paragraph from which the information is derived. You may choose a paragraph more than once. Each paragraph is marked with a letter.**

_____ (1) Music is to him a reliever to sensory overload.

_____ (2) She entered Miss America competition to prove autistic people on a spectrum of low-functioning can fit well in the society.

_____ (3) Not every person likes her in terms of her singing and appearance.

_____ (4) She was too much worried that the public would tease her being a fashion model.

_____ (5) She is highly esteemed by the university she is working for.

_____ (6) Music helps him learn how to better focus.

_____ (7) She has contributed a great deal to the animal sciences.

_____ (8) Her album sold like hot cakes after her performance on Britain's Got Talent.

_____ (9) She finds having her Asperger's syndrome known will make it easier for the public to better understand her.

_____ (10) People in her times did not fully understand autism.

Susan Boyle

A）In 2009，a shy, 47-year-old Scottish woman touched the world with her breathtaking rendition of *Les Misérables'* "I Dreamed A Dream" on Britain's Got Talent. After the performance，Susan Boyle catapulted into a singing sensation，selling more than 14 million records worldwide.

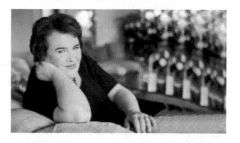

B）This Scottish singer was unknown when she first got on stage to perform on Britain's Got Talent. Her somewhat frumpy appearance and coarse accent did not prepare audiences for the magnificence of her voice. It's safe to say public reception to the singer has been mixed.

C）On the one hand，her voice is incredible；no one can dispute that. On the other，there have been headlines like："Susan Boyle has Asperger's — not brain damage." Last week，she revealed to *The Observer* that she was diagnosed with Asperger syndrome by a Scottish specialist — a revelation that she calls "a relief".

D）"Asperger's doesn't define me. It's a condition that I have to live with and work through，but I feel more relaxed about myself," she said in the interview. "People will have a greater understanding of who I am and why I do the things I do."

James Durbin

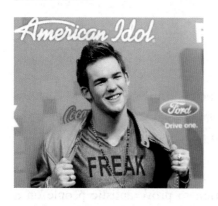

E）The American Idol alum（from season 10），who recently released his new single，"Parachute"，was first diagnosed with Asperger syndrome and Tourette syndrome at age 10. "Right around the time when I was diagnosed，I got a hand-me-down guitar with a chord book and a cheap busted tuner," Durbin told Autism Speaks last month. "I think music is like medicine and can be a benefit for anyone no matter what genre. There's just so much you can learn. It's all about focus and for me，not only on the autism spectrum but also the Tourette's spectrum，focus was something I needed help with. Music is my focus."

F）Music also became a way for Durbin to cope with bullying growing up. "Throughout this process，I figured out that no matter how bad of a day I had at school，I could come home and create my own world within the music," he wrote on CNN. "I could make the music as happy or as sad as I wanted it to be. I used the pain from being bullied to transform me into who I was meant to be."

Temple Grandin

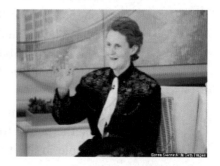

G）Temple Grandin is a professor of animal sciences at Colorado State University，which calls her "the most accomplished and well-known adult with autism in the world". According to her website, Grandin didn't speak until she was three and a half years old, "communicating her frustration instead by screaming, peeping and humming". After receiving a diagnosis of autism, her parents were told she should be institutionalized. She wrote in her book, *Emergence: Labeled Autistic*:

> I have read enough to know that there are still many parents, and yes, professionals too, who believe that "once autistic, always autistic". This dictum has meant sad and sorry lives for many children diagnosed, as I was in early life, as autistic. To these people, it is incomprehensible that the characteristics of autism can be modified and controlled. However, I feel strongly that I am living proof that they can.

H) In addition to her work in the animal sciences (among her other accomplishments, Grandin developed corrals to improve quality of life for cattle), she has become an outspoken advocate in the autism community. In 2010, TIME named her one of the 100 most influential people in the world, and HBO produced a biopic based on her life called *Temple Grandin*, starring Claire Danes as the title character.

Alexis Wineman

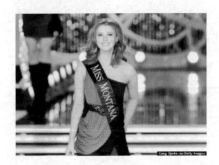

I) Earlier this year, Miss Montana became the first Miss America contestant with autism to compete in the pageant. At age 11, Wineman was diagnosed with pervasive development disorder, CNN reported.

J) "My path may not be one that another person would choose, but I challenged myself to enter the Miss America competition because it seemed like the peak to my own personal Everest," she wrote for CNN in January. "It also seemed kind of ironic: a girl who was told she was different and considered an outcast by many, in the nation's biggest beauty pageant."

K) She reached the top 15 in the competition, and won the America's Choice Award, according to CNN, for garnering the most online viewer votes. "So many people expect autistic people to all be the same — that it's a brain disorder so we can't function in society," she told *TIME*. "I want people to realize there's a whole spectrum of people who live with autism. There are high-functioning people and low-functioning people."

Heather Kuzmich

L) When America's Next Top Model cycle nine began in 2007, the audience met 21-year-old Heather Kuzmich, who was diagnosed with Asperger syndrome. "It was a point in my life where I was thinking either Asperger's was going to define me or I was going to be able to work around it," Kuzmich

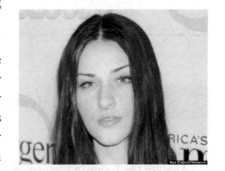

told *The New York Times* of her decision to join the competition show. "At first I was really worried people would laugh at me because I was so very awkward. I got the exact opposite."

M) The contestant finished in fifth place, and was voted as the viewer favorite eight weeks in a row. "I was at the bottom of the totem pole," she told *People* about her time growing up. "I wanted to be a role model for girls who aren't the most popular and are picked on."

2. Read the following statements. Decide to what extent you agree or disagree with each statement, and write your own pros or cons in the box, then set your rational viewpoint and the reasons.

(1) Autistic children should be institutionalized once they are diagnosed autistic.

(2) Autism stops you from living a fulfilling life.

(3) Not all autism diagnoses are precise and there is no exact black-and-white dividing line between normal and autistic children.

(4) We should leave autistic children at home as they are often bullied by others and are socially awkward.

(5) Autistic people need to live with their family.

(6) Early intervention makes no difference for children with autism.

Pros	Cons

VII. Outcome Sentence Analysis and Essay Writing

1. Sentence-structure Analysis
Analyze the following sentences and draw a tree-structure.

(1) There is often nothing about how people with ASD look that sets them apart from other people, but people with ASD may communicate, interact, behave, and learn in ways that are different from most other people.

(2) This report, moreover, was based on a survey of around 3,000 families selected by schools, nonprofits, and other organizations supporting those with autism, which are more likely to be actively searching for jobs for their children.

(3) The training program, launched by the central Hongkou District in 2017, has allowed Cai and 14 other students with special needs to attend Shanghai Nanhu Vocational School, where they have been learning the skills required to work in the hospitality sector.

(4) Spleen *qi* deficiency and kidney essence deficiency are central to the pathology of autism, the former affecting food intake (no interest in food, or an excessive hunger), while the latter will result in poor mental development.

(5) Although alternative autism treatment such as tongue acupuncture and dietary changes should still be viewed as a complementary approach, these exciting early findings stand as an innovative starting point for a new system of autism treatment.

2. Essay writing
   A. Reading for Writing
   Please read the following passage, underlining the useful information considering the following questions.
   (1) What are the major challenges interacting with people diagnosed with autism spectrum disorder?
   (2) How can we build positive relationships with them?

Best Communication Practices for Interacting with People with Autism

Everyone has different strengths, interests, needs and challenges. Just like with any other friend, colleague or acquaintance, learning these are the first step to positive relationships and communication.

People with autism bring new perspectives and ideas, enriching our communities and workplaces with their gifts inspired from seeing the world in different ways. With 1 in 59 American children now diagnosed with some form of autism, if you think you don't know anyone with autism you might be wrong. Being part of the wider community and developing relationships benefits everyone.

We offer these tips and insights to achieve positive relationships and community, understanding more about what being on the autism spectrum means. Depending on the age and ability of the individual you may adapt different communication strategies and accommodations. These techniques are good to use with anyone, regardless of whether they are neurotypical or have ASD. Be respectful, ask what the person prefers, likes and needs.

Ways to Build Relationships and Rapport

- Be patient while having a conversation, giving the person time to answer.
- Always strive to be encouraging and compassionate.
- Learn about their favorite interests, games or hobbies and try to find common ones.
- Be aware of the tendency by people with ASD to speak at length about their favorite topics which may require some gentle prompting or redirection.
- Sustaining conversation can also be challenging. You can support them by offering choices, suggesting topics or bridging the conversation to a topic you know they can discuss.
- Offer concise directions or clear choices. For example, "Would you like to take a walk or ride our bikes?
- Provide specific praise such as "I liked the way you waited for me before leaving the room" instead of a vague "good job" so they understand what behavior you are seeking from them.
- To make your own communication clearer, share with the individual what you want them to do rather than what you don't want them to do (i. e. Instead of saying "don't run, ' it's better to say "please walk in the hall.")
- Don't be offended by lack of eye contact, motor tics or a lack of understanding personal boundaries. These are common challenges for someone with ASD.
- Understand that people with ASD like routines and schedules.
- People with autism tend to think literally, so it is best to avoid idioms and slang.

Pointers to help people with ASD if they get off topic or spend too much time on a topic

- Gentle nudge or prompt to get back on topic such as, What were we talking about again? Or redirect them by bringing up the topic you were originally discussing like, Where should we go for lunch? It sounds like you love Chinese Food, how about XYZ place at 11:45 am? (ideally somewhere not too loud or at crowded time)

- So to summarize, our next steps are XYZ, your part will be this and it will be due by x date. Does that seem to cover what we discussed?
- In a kind yet concrete way, say, I hear you really like talking about dinosaurs, but I am not really interested in that and don't want to talk about it anymore, can we talk about something we are both interested in? Then suggest something that you have in common or could such as favorite movies or food.

Boundary Issues

Social communication can be challenging for people with ASD. They may have different perceptions of spheres of social norms for different types of people. For example, understanding that a teacher or supervisor is not equated with a social friend. Or the difference between a friend and a friendly acquaintance. They may not realize the appropriate amount of personal space to give people. People with autism tend to be more literal so it's helpful to offer them gentle but direct guidance in a kind voice.

If you need to help someone with boundary issues:

- If they seem to stand too close to you, be kind but gently direct. For example, you could say could you please stand about this far apart from me when we're talking? Thanks so much. (You can raise your arm a little to give an idea of how far apart you mean.)
- If the person touches your hair, hugs you inappropriately or similar physical interaction, you can start by moving away out of reach. If it is persistent or bothersome, ask the person to stop. You could also distract them by redirecting them to move their attention to something else like an activity. You can also model the physical distance and appropriate place for your own hands at your sides, in your pocket, arms folded and the like.
- If the person shares personal information you're not comfortable with because you're not a friend or that close to them, try to change the subject to something more appropriate. If that doesn't work, you can gently tell them that topic is a little too personal.

Communication Style

Provide options for how the person prefers to communicate, whether texting on phone, emailing or face to face conversation. Don't assume everyone wants to communicate in the exact same way. Making the purpose or reason for the communication clear (i.e. in college is it social or class project) helps the person with ASD prepare and sets expectations.

People with ASD do well with clarity and structure. However it doesn't need to be formal. An agenda is not necessary, just sharing the topic like, we're going to meet to plan logistics for a specific event.

Be aware that some people have more limited abilities or preferences with communication modes so may need to use nonverbal approaches whether picture schedules, tablets, gesturing or picture exchange systems.

Managing Sensory Issues

People with ASD may have sensory challenges with touch, sound, light, smell or taste more intensely than neurotypical people. You can be helpful and sensitive to them by thinking about loud sounds, bright lights, strong smells and food issues that might be most difficult for your friend or colleague with ASD.

For meetings or business interactions, think about how to be considerate to their needs. For example, avoid restaurants or meeting locations that have intense sensory experiences. Minimize distractions by choosing a quiet, uncluttered location which as a side benefit may help your team focus better. Could look at it as providing soothing, peaceful and zen/meditation like vs the gamified colorful bright vibrant places.

When overstimulated a person with ASD may use different self soothing strategies including leaving the room or area to avoid a meltdown or shutdown. Or they may just have a difficult time focusing and doing their best.

Consider having sensory friendly meeting areas or classrooms, for example with dimmed lights, comfy chairs, limited distractions in the room, neutral colors.

For Those Who Are More Impacted on the Spectrum, Nonverbal or Need Extra Assistance

With people who are more impacted, they will have higher needs in areas such as communication and sensory issues and will need more extensive support in daily living. However, being nonverbal does not necessarily mean higher impacted. Don't presume a person's intellectual capacity based on their being low-verbal or nonverbal.

- Pause after giving directions to allow the person to process the verbal information.
- Offer to provide simply worded written directions or a checklist for routine or novel tasks.
- Give the person choices in the conversation (i. e. "Would you like a sandwich or pizza?").
- Questions should be worded to only provide acceptable options when possible. For example, if a boss says, "Would you like to join us in this meeting?" the individual with ASD saying "no" and returning to their desk is a potential response. This is because a command is being worded as a question. In this case, instead, say, "Please come with us for a meeting in the conference room at 10:00 am." (You may need to come get them depending on their level of functioning.)
- Have the person repeat important information to confirm understanding (i. e. Ask, "Where are we going?" after you've shared that information).
- Use pictures or drawings to help the person communicate (i. e. pictures of food or activity choices).
- Visual schedules in which you provide a photo or graphic to designate different activities planned can also be helpful.
- Although some people can carry on conversations that last for hours, some individuals may only be able to answer a single question, or engage in a conversation for 5 minutes. In these situations, building in breaks for the individual can be productive and help them stay calmer and more focused.

If Someone Is Nonverbal

- Ask the individual or their caregiver how they prefer to communicate.
- Learn what assistive devices or techniques they may use. For example, visual schedule, iPad apps, text-to-speech or other voice assistant apps in which person touches something on their device to speak for them.
- Always look at the individual who you are trying to communicate with, not their caregiver. If you were using a translator for a person speaking a different language you would look at the person you want to communicate with, not the translator.
- Pair your verbal communication with gestures (point to where you want them to hang their coat or nod your head yes to confirm a response).
- If using an assistive device, give them enough time to type in their responses.
- Don't talk about them in front of them like they aren't there.
- Always face them when talking to them even if they don't appear to be paying attention.
- Always communicate what you are doing even if you don't think they understand.

How to Be a Friend to Someone with ASD

The best way to be supportive and develop a good relationship with anyone is by asking how you can be a good friend, colleague, etc. So don't be afraid to ask your friend with ASD, "How can I be a better friend?"

In addition to the tips above, here are some suggestions for being a good friend.

- Listen and don't be quick to give an answer or response when spending time with your friend with ASD. Simply be there to give a listening ear. You may have to wait longer for a response or possibly weed through a lengthy explanation, but you will learn something new in the end.
- Support your friend if they ask for help. Be sensitive to what they want and need, not just how you think they should improve or behave.
- Try not to talk over or about them when others are around.
- Help them work on social skills by trying to engage them in conversations with yourself and others.
- Find discrete ways to give social hints. Build up their confidence in the same way that you would support any other friend in a challenging situation.
- Try not to jump in and make choices for your friend in a social situation.
- Thinking about when you are going to get together with a friend is important. Preventing uncomfortable situations is far easier than dealing with them once they happen. Instead of heading to your favorite brunch spot at 11:00 a.m. on a Sunday morning, try going after the rush at 2:00 p.m. or if you know there's going to be a long line or wait somewhere, plan to arrive early (or late) to avoid the crowds.

B. Writing

Please write a 200-word essay considering the following questions:

1. What are the major challenges in interacting with people diagnosed with autism spectrum disorder?
2. How can we build positive relationships with them?

Unit 4
Precision Medicine

Read the web page. Then answer the questions orally.

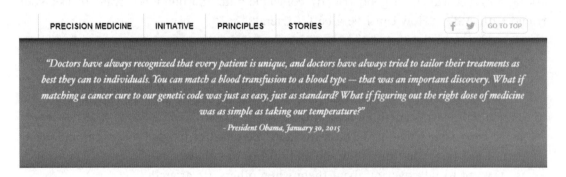

| PRECISION MEDICINE | INITIATIVE | PRINCIPLES | STORIES |

"Doctors have always recognized that every patient is unique, and doctors have always tried to tailor their treatments as best they can to individuals. You can match a blood transfusion to a blood type — that was an important discovery. What if matching a cancer cure to our genetic code was just as easy, just as standard? What if figuring out the right dose of medicine was as simple as taking our temperature?"

- President Obama, January 30, 2015

So what is Precision Medicine?

It's health care tailored to you.

In his 2015 State of the Union address, President Obama announced that he's launching the Precision Medicine Initiative — a bold new research effort to revolutionize how we improve health and treat disease.

Until now, most medical treatments have been designed for the "average patient". As a result of this "one-size-fits-all" approach, treatments can be very successful for some patients but not for others. Precision Medicine, on the other hand, is an innovative approach that takes into account individual differences in people's genes, environments, and lifestyles. It gives medical professionals the resources they need to target the specific treatments of the illnesses we encounter, further develops our scientific and medical research, and keeps our families healthier.

Advances in Precision Medicine have already led to powerful new discoveries and several new treatments that are tailored to specific characteristics, such as a person's genetic makeup, or the genetic profile of an individual's tumor. This is helping transform the way we can treat diseases such as cancer: Patients with breast, lung, and colorectal cancers, as well as melanomas and leukemias, for instance, routinely undergo molecular testing as part of patient care, enabling physicians to select treatments that improve chances of survival and reduce exposure to adverse effects.

And we're committed to protecting your privacy every step of the way. The White House is working with the Department of Health and Human Services and other federal agencies to solicit input from patient groups, bioethicists, privacy and civil liberties advocates, technologists, and other experts, to help identify and address any legal and technical issues related to the privacy and security of data in the context of Precision Medicine.

precision [prɪˈsɪʒən]	*n.* the quality of being exact, accurate and careful 精确;准确;细致
initiative [ɪˈnɪʃɪətɪv]	*n.* a new plan for dealing with a particular problem or for achieving a particular purpose 倡议;新方案
tumor [ˈtjuːmə(r)]	*n.* an abnormal new mass of tissue that serves no purpose 肿瘤
colorectal [ˌkəʊləˈrektəl]	*adj.* relating to or affecting the colon and the rectum 结肠直肠的
adverse [ˈædvɜːs]	*adj.* negative and unpleasant 不利的;有害的

(1) What is "one-size-fits-all" approach?

_____

(2) What will be taken into account in precision medicine?

_____

(3) How does precision medicine help transform the way we treat diseases?

_____

(4) How can we ensure patients' privacy and security in the context of precision medicine?

_____

II. Watching-in Precision Public Health

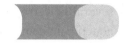

1. View the video clips. Match the photos (A – D) to the dialogues (1 – 4). Then answer the following questions.

A.

Big Data
Consumer Monitoring
Genetic Sequencing

B.

C.

D.

Precision
Public Health
2016

Video clip 1: _____   Video clip 2: _____
Video clip 3: _____   Video clip 4: _____

(1) Why in the area of Ethiopia, parents delay picking the names for their new babies by a month or more according to video 1?

_____

(2) What are the side effects in a normal treatment of cancer according to video 2?

_____

(3) How can we applied a precision public health approach in certain areas of Africa according to video 3?

_____

(4) What can we expect if we apply the precision public health according to video 4?

_____
_____

2. View the video clips again. Fill in the blanks to complete the sentences which can help you get the gist of the content.

(1)

Speaker:

I travel a lot and I see a lot. But it took me by surprise to learn in an area of Ethiopia, parents delay picking the names for their new babies by a month or more.

They're afraid their baby will die. And this loss might be a little more bearable without a name. A face without a name might help them feel just a little less 1) _____ .

How can it be that 2.6 million babies die around the world before they're even one month old? 2.6 million. That's the 2) _____ of Vancouver. And the shocking thing is: Why? In too many cases, we simply don't know.

So our first step in restoring the dreams of those parents is to answer the question: Why are babies dying?

So today, I want to talk about a new approach, an approach that I feel will not only help us know why babies are dying, but is beginning to completely 3) _____ the whole field of global health. It's called "Precision Public Health".

(2)

Speaker:

For me, precision medicine comes from a very special place. I trained as a cancer doctor, an oncologist. I got into it because I wanted to help people feel better. But too often my treatments made them feel 1) _____ .

And so the side effects that you're all very familiar with — hair loss, being sick to your stomach, having a suppressed immune system, so infection was a constant threat — were always 2) _____ us.

I got to work on a new approach for breast cancer patients that could do a better job of telling the healthy cells from the unhealthy or cancer cells. It's a drug called Herceptin. And what Herceptin allowed us to do is to 3) _____ target HER2-positive breast cancer, at the time, the scariest form of breast cancer. And that precision let us hit hard the cancer cells, while sparing and being more gentle on the normal cells ... so much so that today, we're harnessing all those tools — big data, consumer 4) _____ , gene sequencing and more — to tackle a broad variety of diseases. That's allowing us to target individuals with the right 5) _____ at the right time.

(3)

Speaker：

Let's go back to the 2.6 million babies who die before they're one month old. Here's the problem：we just don't know. It may seem unbelievable，but the way we figure out the causes of infant 1) _____ in those countries with the highest infant mortality is a conversation with mom.

And even worse — it's not that helpful，because we might know there was a fever or vomiting，but we don't know why. So in the 2) _____ of knowing that knowledge, we cannot prevent that mom，that family，or other families in that community from suffering the same tragedy.

But what if we applied a precision public health approach?

And that's the point：Once we know，we can bring the right 3) _____ to the right population in the right places to save lives.

I have no doubt that a precision public health approach can help our world achieve our 15-year goal. And that would translate into a million babies' lives saved every single year. One million babies every single year.

(4)

Speaker：

A much more powerful approach to public health — imagine what might be possible. Why couldn't we more effectively tackle malnutrition? Why wouldn't we prevent cervical cancer in women? And why not eradicate malaria?

So，you know，I live in two different worlds，one world populated by scientists，and another world populated by public health professionals. The 1) _____ of precision public health is to bring these two worlds together. But you know，we all live in two worlds：the rich world and the poor world. And what I'm most excited about about precision public health is 2) _____ these two worlds. Every day in the rich world，we're bringing incredible talent and tools — everything at our disposal — to precisely target diseases in ways I never imagined would be possible. Surely，we can tap into that kind of talent and tools to stop babies dying in the poor world. If we did，then every parent would have the 3) _____ to name their child the moment that child is born，daring to dream that that child's life will be measured in decades，not days.

oncologist [ɒŋˈkɒlədʒɪst]	*n.* the scientific study of and treatment of tumour in the body 肿瘤学
harness [ˈhɑːnɪs]	*v.* to control and use the force or strength of sth to produce power or to achieve sth 控制，利用（以产生能量等）
tackle [ˈtækl]	*v.* to try to deal with a difficult problem 应付，解决（难题或局面）
cervical [ˈsɜːvɪkəl]	*adj.* connected with the cervix 子宫颈的
eradicate [ɪˈrædɪkeɪt]	*v.* to destroy or get rid of sth completely，especially sth bad 根除；消灭；杜绝
malaria [məˈleərɪə]	*n.* a disease that causes fever and shivering（＝shaking of the body）caused by the bite of some types of mosquito 疟疾
disposal [dɪˈspəʊzəl]	*n.* the act of getting rid of sth 去掉；清除；处理

III. Leading-in Defining Precision Medicine

1. **View a video clip and answer the questions.**
   (1) According to the video，what is precision medicine?
   _____
   _____

   (2) What is the significance of precision medicine according to the video?
   _____
   _____

2. **Read the following passage and answer these questions.**
   (1) What does precision medicine take into account?
   _____
   _____

   (2) What factors may influence our health besides genes?
   _____
   _____

   (3) What efforts have been made to deal with a deluge of new sequence data hitting the networks each day?
   _____
   _____

（4）What are the additional approaches to precision medicine beyond the genome?

_____

_____

（5）What are the other purposes of precision medicine besides treating diseases?

_____

_____

_____

Passage A

Precision Medicine

Right now, most medical treatments are designed for the average patient. Precision medicine, on the other hand, matches each patient with the treatment that will work best for them. Also called personalized medicine or individualized medicine, precision medicine takes individual variation into account: variation in our genes, environment, lifestyle, and even in the microscopic organisms that are living inside of us.

Genes + Environment = Health Status

At the center of precision medicine are efforts to understand how variations in our genes influence our health. Just like genetic variations contribute to physical characteristics like height and hair color, they also influence our likelihood of getting certain diseases. Some genetic variations protect us from disease, and some make us more susceptible.

Genetic variations also influence how we respond to medications and other interventions. For instance, it is crucial to know a person's blood type before giving them a transfusion. And understanding individual variations in the enzymes that process drugs can help a doctor prescribe the right dose of the right medication.

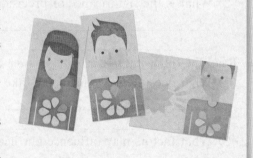

But as anyone who knows identical twins can tell you, we are more than a collection of genes. Factors from the environment — including our physical surroundings, our diet, and our lifestyle — also influence our health. For example, even if someone inherits genetic variations that make them susceptible to skin cancer, they can decrease their chances of getting cancer by protecting themselves from the sun. Precision medicine involves understanding how factors from the environment interact with genetic variations to influence health. When combined with information about a person's environment, genetic information becomes even more powerful.

Medicine in the Genomic Age

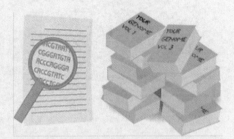

Each person's genome contains about 6 billion letters of DNA code. Contained within that code are the instructions for building all of the proteins that make their cells, tissues, and organs function. Some serious health conditions are linked to a single letter of code. Others are linked to combinations of more subtle variations spread throughout the genome.

There has been a lot of buzz lately about the plummeting cost and skyrocketing speed of DNA sequencing. In 2001, a human genome cost about $100 million to sequence. 2014 began with an announcement of a new machine that could sequence 16 human genomes in 3 days at a cost of about $1,000 per genome. What this means for patients is that whole-genome sequencing is now as affordable as many routine medical tests, and it's becoming increasingly available.

For no more than the cost of an MRI scan, patients will be able to obtain their entire genomic sequence, a resource that will continue to inform medical decisions for them over the course of their lifetime.

Sequencing even one human genome generates a lot of information — about 200 gigabytes of raw data — and it takes some serious computational power to chug through it. With a deluge of new sequence data hitting the networks each day, efforts have turned to developing tools and systems for storing, sharing, and analyzing this data on a large scale. With these tools, researchers can analyze genomic information from large numbers of people — some with disease and others without. It may seem counterintuitive, but the more genomic information your doctors understand about everybody else, the better equipped they are to offer individualized care to you.

Beyond the Genome

Understanding how genetic variations contribute to health is just one aspect of precision medicine. While the genome is set for life, the expression of our genes fluctuates over time and in response to the environment. Additional approaches to precision medicine involve measuring levels of proteins, RNAs, or metabolic products. Along with genomics, proteomics, epigenomics, and metabolomics can help inform medical choices for individual patients.

The field also incorporates what we are learning about the microbes that live in and on our bodies and how they can be manipulated to influence health and disease. It combines the latest in stem cell science with 3D printing technology to build replacement skin, blood vessels, and bones. It includes techniques for engineering a patient's own immune cells to attack cancer and other diseases, and computer algorithms for building customized diets for diabetic patients.

Beyond treating disease, precision medicine includes approaches to diagnostics, prevention, and screening:

◇ Methods for identifying those who are at risk before disease strikes；

◇ Analytical tools for predicting which prevention strategies will work best for which patients；

◇ Screening methods that can identify early signs of disease before symptoms emerge；

◇ Diagnostic methods for identifying subtypes of disease that may look the same on the surface but respond very differently to treatment；

◇ Tests that can identify disease carrier status for prospective parents；

◇ Devices for managing diseases and for tracking and guiding recovery.

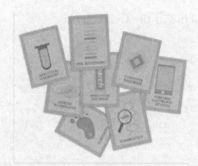

Precision medicine combines the best of basic research and modern technology, leveraging recent gains not only in DNA sequencing and analysis, but also in the areas of genetic technology, protein biochemistry, cancer research, personal electronic devices, search engine software, computer chip manufacturing, and much more.

microscopic [ˌmaɪkrə'skɒpɪk]	*adj*. extremely small and difficult or impossible to see without a microscope 极小的；微小的；需用显微镜观察的
susceptible [sə'septəbl]	*adj*. very likely to be influenced，harmed or affected by sb/sth 易受影响(或伤害等)的；敏感；过敏
enzyme ['enzaɪm]	*n*. a substance，produced by all living things, which helps a chemical change happen or happen more quickly, without being changed itself 酶
inherit [ɪn'herɪt]	*v*. to have qualities, physical features, etc. that are similar to those of your parents, grandparents, etc. 经遗传获得(品质、身体特征等)
buzz [bʌz]	*v*. a strong feeling of pleasure, excitement or achievement (愉快、兴奋或成就的强烈情感)
plummet ['plʌmɪt]	*v*. to fall suddenly and quickly from a high level or position 暴跌；速降
skyrocket ['skaɪˌrɒkɪt]	*v*. (of prices, etc.) to rise quickly to a very high level 飞涨；猛涨

sequence [ˈsiːkwəns]	*v.* to identify the order in which a set of genes or parts of molecules are arranged 测定(整套基因或分子成分的)序列
gigabyte [ˈdʒɪɡəbaɪt]	*n.* a unit of computer memory, equal to 10^9 (or about a billion) bytes 十亿字节;吉字节;千兆字节
chug [tʃʌg]	*v.* to make slow but steady progress 缓慢而稳步地进展
counterintuitive [ˌkaʊntərɪnˈtjuːɪtɪv]	*adj.* contrary to what common sense would suggest 违反直觉的
fluctuate [ˈflʌktjʊeɪt]	*v.* to change frequently in size, amount, quality, etc., especially from one extreme to another 波动;起伏不定
RNA	*abbr.* ribonucleic acid, a chemical present in all living cells; like DNA it is a type of nucleic acid 核糖核酸
genomics [dʒiːˈnəʊmɪks]	*n.* the branch of genetics that studies organisms in terms of their genomes (their full DNA sequences) 基因组学
proteomics [ˌprəʊtɪˈɒmɪks]	*n.* the branch of genetics that studies the full set of proteins encoded by a genome 蛋白质组学
epigenomics [ˌepɪdʒɪˈnɒmɪks]	*n.* the study of the epigenome, which is a multitude of chemical compounds that direct the functioning genome as a whole 表观基因组学
metabolomics [ˌmetəbəˈlɒmɪks]	*n.* a new branch in analytical biochemistry that is related to metabolism 代谢组学
algorithm [ˈælɡərɪðəm]	*n.* a set of rules that must be followed when solving a particular problem 算法;计算程序
screening [ˈskriːnɪŋ]	*n.* the testing or examining of a large number of people or things for disease, faults, etc. 筛查

3. **Match each of the terms listed below with the numbered definition. Write the letter in the space provided.**

A. genome	E. mutation	I. microbiome
B. targeted therapy	F. metabolomics	J. cellular analysis
C. molecule	G. clinical trial	K. sequence
D. proteomics	H. imaging	L. customize

(1) _____: obtaining pictures of the interior of the body

(2) _____: the study of all the metabolites present in cells, tissues and organs

(3) _____: the action of change in the cells of a living thing producing a new quality in the material or parts of the body

(4) _____: the smallest part of any substance that can exist without losing its own chemical nature, consisting of one or more atoms

(5) _____: the order in which things or events follow one another

(6) _____: the collection of microorganisms in or on the body

(7) _____: a medical treatment that blocks the growth of cancer cells by interfering with specific targeted molecules needed for carcinogenesis and tumor growth, rather than by simply interfering with all rapidly dividing cells

(8) _____: the branch of biochemistry concerned with the structure and analysis of the proteins occurring in living organisms

(9) _____: the ordering of genes in a haploid set of chromosomes of a particular organism

(10) _____: an investigation of cellular function

(11) _____: to make or change something according to the buyer's or user's needs

(12) _____: a rigorously controlled test of a new drug or a new invasive medical device on human subjects

IV. Critical Reading Further Reading on Precision Medicine

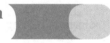

1. History of Precision Medicine

Read the following passage and complete the exercises that follow.

A. Fill in the blanks to complete the table.

Year	Event
1871	Fredrich Meischer identified (1)_____, now known as (2)_____.
(3)_____	Frederick Sanger developed first DNA sequencing method.
(4)_____	First draft of the (5)_____ was released.
2003	(6)_____ was completed.
2007	New (7)_____ technology developed, increasing capability (8)_____.
(9)_____	President Obama launched (10)_____.

B. Judge whether the following statements are true (T) or false (F).

_____ (1) The prospect of applying precision medicine broadly has been greatly improved by the recent development of large-scale biologic databases.

_____ (2) The long-term aim of Obama's Precision Medicine Initiative is to generate knowledge applicable to the whole range of health and disease.

_____ (3) Targeted therapies focus on where the cancer develops in the body.

_____ (4) 3D drugs can be printed based on a patient's personalized information.

_____ (5) China has been a leader in the precision medicine field.

Passage B

History of Precision Medicine: Where Science Meets Technology

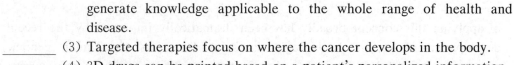

Scientific Breakthroughs

1871 Fredrich Meischer identifies "nuclein", now known as DNA, in the nucleus of cells.

1953 Watson and Crick determine the double-helix structure of DNA.

1977 Frederick Sanger develops the first DNA sequencing method.

1990 Human genome project is launched with goal of 15 years.

2001 First draft of the human genome is released.

2002 Mouse is the first mammal to have genome sequenced.

2003 Human Genome Project is completed

2007 New gene sequencing technology developed, increasing capability 70-fold

2008 1,000 genomes project is launched.

2012 Encode Study publishes 30 papers of results of active sites in genome hit.
    begins to focus on data warehousing and analytics solutions

State of Hit/ Medical Technology

1960s Computers begin to give rise to shared accounting systems at hospitals.

1970s Computers are small enough to have departmental systems in hospitals.

1980s Integrated financial and clinical systems begin to emerge, as well as managed care financial and administrative systems.

1990s Integrated financial and clinical systems begin to emerge, as well as managed care financial and administrative systems.

2000s Emergence of commercial, real-time clinical decision support

2010 1,000 genomes project results are published.
2013 President Obama launches the Precision Medicine Initiative.

Obama's Precision Medicine Initiative

"Tonight, I'm launching a new Precision Medicine Initiative to bring us closer to curing diseases like cancer and diabetes — and to give all of us access to the personalized information we need to keep ourselves and our families healthier."

— President Barack Obama, State of the Union Address, January 20, 2015

President Obama has long expressed a strong conviction that science offers great potential for improving health. In 2015, he announced a research initiative that aims to accelerate progress toward a new era of precision medicine.

The concept of precision medicine — prevention and treatment strategies that take individual variability into account — is not new; blood typing, for instance, has been used to guide blood transfusions for more than a century. But the prospect of applying this concept broadly has been dramatically improved by the recent development of large-scale biologic databases (such as the human genome sequence), powerful methods for characterizing patients (such as proteomics, metabolomics, genomics, diverse cellular assays, and even mobile health technology), and computational tools for analyzing large sets of data. What is needed now is a broad research program to encourage creative approaches to precision medicine, test them rigorously, and ultimately use them to build the evidence base needed to guide clinical practice.

The proposed initiative has two main components: a near-term focus on cancers and a longer-term aim to generate knowledge applicable to the whole range of health and disease. Both components are within our reach because of advances in basic research, including molecular biology, genomics, and bioinformatics. Furthermore, the initiative taps into converging trends of increased connectivity through social media and mobile devices.

Understanding Precision Medicine in Cancer Treatment

The hope of precision medicine is that treatments will one day be tailored to the changes in each person's cancer. Scientists see a future when patients will receive drugs that their tumors are most likely to respond to and will be spared from receiving drugs that are not likely to help. Research studies are going on now to test whether treating patients with drugs that target the cancer-causing genetic changes in their tumors, no matter where the cancer develops in the body, will help them. Many of these drugs are known as targeted therapies.

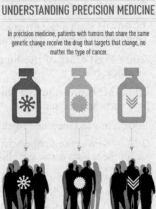

UNDERSTANDING PRECISION MEDICINE

In precision medicine, patients with tumors that share the same genetic change receive the drug that targets that change, no matter the type of cancer.

Targeted therapy is the foundation of precision medicine. It is a type of cancer treatment that targets the changes in cancer cells that help them grow, divide, and spread. As researchers learn more about the cell changes that drive cancer, they are better able to design promising therapies that target these changes or block their effects.

Most targeted therapies are either small-molecule drugs or monoclonal antibodies. Small-molecule drugs are small enough to enter cells easily, so they are used for targets that are inside cells. Monoclonal antibodies are drugs that are not able to enter cells easily. Instead, they attach to specific targets on the outer surface of cancer cells.

Most targeted therapies help treat cancer by interfering with specific proteins that help tumors grow and spread throughout the body. They treat cancer in many different ways. They can help the immune system destroy cancer cells, stop cancer cells from growing, deliver cell-killing substances to cancer cells and cause cancer cell death. However, targeted therapies do have some drawbacks: 1) Cancer cells can become resistant to them. For this reason, targeted therapies may work best when used with other targeted therapies or with other cancer treatments, such as chemotherapy and radiation. 2) Drugs for some targets are hard to develop. Reasons include the target's structure, the target's function in the cell, or both.

Precision Medicine via 3D Printed Drugs

In April of 2015 the FDA approved its first ever 3D printed pills. Progressing even farther, a team of researchers recently announced the development of a prototype computer algorithm that can print 3D drugs with personalized information. This means drugs can be printed based on a patient's weight, race, gender, and other biological characteristics — a true form of "personalized medicine".

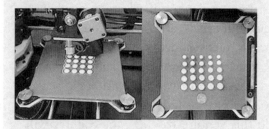

A 3D printer and a customizable dosing algorithm can push pharmaceuticals to the personalized medicine stage. The prototype was unveiled at the American Heart Association Scientific Sessions by Dr. Min Pu, MD, a professor of internal medicine at Wake Forest University in Winston-Salem, North Carolina. Taking input of individual patients' characteristics, the software can calculate the appropriate dosing information that gets sent to the 3D printer, generating fully personalized pills.

A total of 80 3D-printed pills were successfully generated with their algorithm. Doses ranged from 124 mg to 373 mg, with high reproducibility and low variability (standard deviation of 3 – 5 mg).

"Patients are not all the same. The way we react to a drug is dictated in part by our genetics as well as many other individual factors. Currently, pill dosages are dosed based on a 'standard' patient. That's akin to a clothing store only selling suits of three different sizes and expecting a perfect fit for all customers." Dr. Min Pu.

Medicine that adjusts for individual characteristics should theoretically result in increased efficacy and reduced side effects. At least that's the hope. But personalized 3D printing of drugs is not going to replace traditional preformulated drugs any time soon — the customization technology is still in its infancy and the process of 3D printing drugs is not yet cost-effective.

Still, this is one of the earliest studies that marry 3D printing and pharmacogenetics. The resulting product can be truly called "personalized medicine".

Precision Medicine in China

Boiled down to its essence, precision medicine describes the ability to tailor therapies to a patient's individual needs by examining their particular physiology, genome, and environment. The ideal is that individualized treatment will lead to lower costs, fewer side effects, and better outcomes. Precision medicine in China, if not in its infancy, is still a long way from 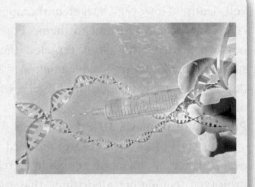 reaching maturity. However, it shows significant promise. The country provides unique opportunities for research, including a varied geography and a large population presenting with many different diseases, both common and rare. Furthermore, the government is clearly a strong proponent of precision medicine, supporting it financially through numerous initiatives and also through policy changes at a national level. This supplement takes a deeper look at precision medicine in China, including associated research undertakings and how it is currently being applied in the diagnosis and treatment of disease, with a particular focus on cancer. There is little doubt that China intends to be a leader in this area, investing both money and resources. Should this venture pay off, the country will be well placed to provide top-quality healthcare for its populace and even to provide advice to other nations with less-advanced health care systems.

diabetes [ˌdaɪə'biːtiːz]	*n.* a disease marked by high levels of sugar in the blood 糖尿病
conviction [kən'vɪkʃən]	*n.* a strong opinion or belief 坚定的看法(或信念)
assay [ə'seɪ]	*n.* the testing of metals and chemicals for quality, often to see how pure they are 含量测定
rigorously ['rɪgərəslɪ]	*adv.* done carefully and with a lot of attention to detail 谨慎的;细致的;彻底的
propose [prəʊ'pəʊz]	*v.* to suggest a plan, an idea, etc. for people to think about and decide on 提议;建议
converge [kən'vɜːdʒ]	*v.* to move towards a place from different directions and meet 汇集;聚集;集中

monoclonal [ˌmɒnəˈkləʊnəl]	*adj.* forming or derived from a single clone 单克隆的
radiation [ˌreɪdɪˈeɪʃn]	*n.* the process in which energy is emitted as particles or waves 辐射；放射线
prototype [ˈprəʊtəʊtaɪp]	*n.* the first design of sth from which other forms are copied or developed 原型；雏形；最初形态
unveil [ˌʌnˈveɪl]	*v.* to show or introduce a new plan, product, etc. to the public for the first time（首次）展示，介绍，推出；将……公之于众
calculate [ˈkælkjuleɪt]	*v.* to use numbers to find out a total number, amount, distance, etc. 计算，核算；预测，推测
reproducibility [ˌriːprədjʊsəˈbɪlɪtɪ]	*n.* the quality of being reproducible 重复能力，再现性；可复演性
dictate [ˈdɪkteɪt]	*v.* to control or influence how sth happens 支配；摆布；决定
efficacy [ˈefɪkəsɪ]	*n.* the ability of sth, especially a drug or a medical treatment, to produce the results that are wanted（尤指药物或治疗方法的）功效，效验，效力
pharmacogenetics [ˌfɑːməkəʊdʒɪˈnetɪks]	*n.* the branch of genetics that studies the genetically determined variations in responses to drugs in humans or laboratory organisms 遗传药理学，药物反应遗传学
infancy [ˈɪnfənsɪ]	*n.* the early development of sth 初期；初创期
proponent [prəʊˈpəʊnənt]	*n.* a person who supports an idea or course of action 倡导者；支持者；拥护者
venture [ˈventʃə(r)]	*n.* a business project or activity, especially one that involves taking risks（尤指有风险的）企业，商业，经营活动
populace [ˈpɒpjʊləs]	*n.* all the ordinary people of a particular country or area 平民百姓；民众

2. China Leaps Ahead in Precision Medicine

Read the following passage to complete the note-taking table, and then check your understanding.

The country's healthcare AI companies:

(1) Beijing Genomics Institute (BGI)

1) It is already the world's largest _____ of genetic material.

2) It is an example of how China is leading the way in _____ to understand human genetics and biology

(2) iCarbonX

1) It collects data on the _____ of millions of patients and uses __ _____ to formulate the best treatments based on a digital, holistic view of each patient.

2) Its ambition is to build _____ that is a one-stop shop for all things health and wellness.

3) The company announced the establishment of iCarbonX-Israel and the acquisition of _____ _____ .

(3) NextCODE

1) It developed _____ that is used by researchers around the world, launched a partnership with Huawei in 2016.

2) The platform develops _____ required to store and compute the massive amounts of data needed for precision medicine.

3) The company is aiming to develop applications that may give doctors _____ _____ with greater accuracy, and help pharmaceutical companies develop _____ _____ .

(4) Yidu Cloud

1) It's a fast-growing company that is playing an important role in precision medicine and health data-driven projects in China, specializes in _____ .

2) It uses _____ to drive real world data research.

3) The company has already processed the data of _____ by setting up cloud services in participating Chinese hospitals or among groups of hospitals.

Passage C

China Leaps Ahead in Precision Medicine

China is positioning itself as a global leader in precision medicine, the use of a person's genetic information to diagnose and treat diseases. "When it comes to understanding precision medicine, China has an historical advantage because Chinese herbal medicine was always tailored to the individual," says Mao Wen, the World Economic Forum's precision medicine project lead in China. "Now China is trying to apply this principle to many cutting-edge technologies." It is no surprise then that one of the focuses of the Forum's new Centre for the Fourth Industrial Revolution in China will be on advances in precision medicine. (The opening of the new centre will be announced at the Forum's Annual Meeting of the New Champions in Tianjin Sept. 18 - 20.)

China is investing in the scientific research to deeply understand the genetics and biological makeup of people, cutting-edge data collection and analysis tools, and powerful computing capabilities to make discoveries from large quantities of data, says Genya Dana, the head of the Forum's precision medicine project.

And precision medicine needs all three of these things to succeed. In 2016, the government earmarked $9 billion over 15 years to sequence and analyze genomes. That dwarfs the $215 million precision-medicine initiative launched in the US the same year. Nearly 40 countries have their own version of a precision medicine initiative, but China's is the largest, says Dana.

A One-Stop Shop for Health and Wellness

China's population of 1.4 billion — and a government willing and able to encourage the sharing of data — give the country's healthcare AI companies an advantage. Shenzhen's Beijing Genomics Institute (BGI) is already the world's largest sequencer and repository of genetic material, the information on which many precision medicine diagnostics and treatments will be based — an example of how China is leading the way in data collection and analysis tools to understand human genetics and biology, says Dana. The third way China is leading in precision medicine is through the development of computational power and artificial intelligence programs to discover new drugs and treatments and deliver them to the right patients. For example, iCarbonX, a Chinese company founded in 2015, collects data on the genetics, environment and behavior of millions of patients and uses AI and data mining to formulate the best treatments based on a digital, holistic view of each patient. ICarbonX's ambition is to build a consumer-facing AI platform that is a one-stop shop for all things health and wellness — from skincare and nutrition recommendations to genetic analysis — with users unlocking different functionalities based on their level of membership. At the highest tier, users would even be offered health and life insurance.

Touted as the "Google of biotech" when it was launched, iCarbonX was founded by a team that includes former employees of BGI. Wang Jun, the founder and CEO of iCarbonX, had previously cofounded BGI. In addition, the iCarbonX co-founder and chief scientist Li Yingrui also has a background at BGI, where he served as both chief scientist and CEO and continues to be a board member.

Its strong foothold in the genomics industry and a strong reputation in gene sequencing technology helped iCarbonX raise its first round of disclosed funding less than a year after launch — a $154 million Series A backed by the Chinese Internet giant Tencent Holdings, says a report from CB Insights. The report notes that the round was the largest first equity round for a healthcare AI company to date, and resulted in instant unicorn status for iCarbonX, which received a $1 billion valuation. Earlier this month the company announced the establishment of iCarbonX-Israel and the acquisition of Image Vision Technologies, a privately-held Israeli image understanding and artificial intelligence company.

Another startup, WuXi NextCODE, which is developing a global platform for genetic data that is used by researchers around the world, launched a partnership with Huawei in 2016 to develop the cloud computing infrastructure required to store and compute the massive amounts of data needed for precision medicine. The company is aiming to develop applications that may give doctors the ability to diagnose more prevalent illnesses with greater accuracy, and help pharmaceutical companies develop more effective treatments. To that end, it has built partnerships with many of the world's biggest pharmaceutical companies, including Novartis, AbbVie and Bristol-Myers Squibb, as well as medical institutions such as Boston Children's Hospital and Peking Union Medical College Hospital, according to press reports.

A third company, Yidu Cloud, a fast-growing company that is playing an important role in precision medicine and health data-driven projects in China, specializes in big data analytics in healthcare. It uses AI to drive real world data research. The company has already processed the data of over 300 million patients by setting up cloud services in participating Chinese hospitals or among groups of hospitals. It works with medical research institutes to form partnerships with hospitals to use data sets for researching diseases and treatments.

Taking Stock of the Challenges

"The data is not just clinical data from diagnosis and treatment, but is full life cycle data integrated with the health information records inside and outside hospitals," says Yu Dan, the company's chief marketing officer.

Instead of prescribing treatments that have been developed for the average person, the dream is that we will instead take only treatments that we know will work based on who we are and how we live our lives. Instead of a one-size-fits-all approach, medicine would be tailored to you.

But there are several challenges for Chinese companies and companies elsewhere to achieve the dream of personalizing medicine, the Forum's Dana says in a blog post. "Doctors and healthcare providers have to learn new technologies and tools to harness the latest science and complex data to understand their patients and tailor precise treatments," she writes. "They will need the tools to communicate these complex ideas to their patients. Patients will want to know how their sensitive personal data about genetics and biology are protected and how they are being used." Addressing these challenges and ensuring that precision medicine is available to all, and not just a privileged few, will require a great deal more work by scientists, new public-private partnerships, and collaboration with civil society, patients, industry, and policy-makers, say experts. But with high levels of funding and enormous amounts of Big Data, China is leading the way forward.

forum [ˈfɔːrəm]	*n.* a place where people can exchange opinions and ideas on a particular issue; a meeting organized for this purpose 公共讨论场所;论坛;讨论会
tout [taʊt]	*v.* to try to persuade people that sb/sth is important or valuable by praising them/it 标榜;吹捧;吹嘘

3. Lexical chunks and sentence rewriting

A. Substitute the underlined part with the words or expressions you have learned.

(1) Also called personalized medicine or individualized medicine, precision medicine <u>takes individual variation into account</u>: variation in our genes, environment, lifestyle, and even in the microscopic organisms that are living inside of us. (passage A)

Answer:

Also called personalized medicine or individualized medicine, precision medicine _____: variation in our genes, environment, lifestyle, and even in the microscopic organisms that are living inside of us.

(2) For <u>no more than</u> the cost of an MRI scan, patients will be able to obtain their entire genomic sequence, a resource that will continue to inform medical decisions for them over the course of their lifetime. (passage A)

Answer:

For the cost of an MRI scan _____, patients will be able to obtain their entire genomic sequence, a resource that will continue to inform medical decisions for them over the course of their lifetime.

(3) With a deluge of new sequence data hitting the networks each day, efforts have turned to developing tools and systems for storing, sharing, and analyzing this data <u>on a large scale</u>. (passage A)

Answer:

With a deluge of new sequence data hitting the networks each day, efforts have turned to developing tools and systems for storing, sharing, and analyzing this data _____.

(4) <u>Along with</u> genomics, proteomics, epigenomics, and metabolomics can help inform medical choices for individual patients. (passage A)

Answer:

_____ genomics, proteomics, epigenomics, and metabolomics can help inform medical choices for individual patients.

(5) Instead, they <u>attach to</u> specific targets on the outer surface of cancer cells. (passage B)

Answer:

Instead, they _____ specific targets on the outer surface of cancer cells.

(6) A total of 80 3D-printed pills <u>were successfully generated with</u> their algorithm. （passage B）

Answer：

A total of 80 3D-printed pills _____ their algorithm.

(7) Medicine that adjusts for individual characteristics should theoretically <u>result in</u> increased efficacy and reduced side effects. （passage B）

Answer：

Medicine that adjusts for individual characteristics should theoretically _____ increased efficacy and reduced side effects.

(8) Should this venture <u>pay off</u>, the country will be well placed to provide top-quality healthcare for its populace and even to provide advice to other nations with less-advanced health care systems. （passage B）

Answer：

Should this venture _____, the country will be well placed to provide top-quality health care for its populace and even to provide advice to other nations with less-advanced health care systems.

(9) <u>When it comes to</u> understanding precision medicine China has an historical advantage because Chinese herbal medicine was always tailored to the individual. （passage C）

Answer：

_____ understanding precision medicine China has an historical advantage because Chinese herbal medicine was always tailored to the individual.

(10) Nearly 40 countries <u>have their own version of</u> a precision medicine initiative, but China's is the largest. （passage C）

Answer：

Nearly 40 countries _____ a precision medicine initiative, but China's is the largest.

(11) In addition, the iCarbonX co-founder and chief scientist Yingrui Li also has a background at BGI, where he <u>served as</u> both chief scientist and CEO and continues to be a board member. （passage C）

Answer：

In addition, the iCarbonX co-founder and chief scientist Yingrui Li also has a background at BGI, where he _____ both chief scientist and CEO and continues to be a board member.

(12) <u>To that end</u>, it has built partnerships with many of the world's biggest pharmaceutical companies. （passage C）

Answer：

_____, it has built partnerships with many of the world's biggest pharmaceutical companies.

B. Rewrite the following sentences using the academic expressions you have learned in the articles.

(1) This difference is often accompanied with the partial or complete abortion of the reproductive organs.

Lexical chunks: _____

Sentence rewriting: _____

_____

(2) Referring to my conversation with you today, I now enclose an order sheet for hosiery as specified.

Lexical chunks: _____

Sentence rewriting: _____

_____

(3) This paint will adhere to any surface, whether rough or smooth.

Lexical chunks: _____

Sentence rewriting: _____

_____

(4) The setting of mechanical specifications for catalysts should take into consideration the needs of the user.

Lexical chunks: _____

Sentence rewriting: _____

_____

(5) Many companies are expecting flat sales or at most a 1 to 2 percent increase over last year.

Lexical chunks: _____

Sentence rewriting: _____

_____

4. **Bilingual translation**

Put the following into Chinese or vice versa.

A. English-Chinese translation

Learn the following useful expressions by translating the sentences selected from the passages.

(1) on a large scale 大规模地

Excerpt:

With a deluge of new sequence data hitting the networks each day, efforts have turned to developing tools and systems for storing, sharing, and analyzing this data on a large scale.

Translation:

_____

_____

(2) the range of ……的范围

Excerpt:

The proposed initiative has two main components: a near-term focus on cancers and a longer-term aim to generate knowledge applicable to the whole range of health and disease.

Translation：

_____

_____

（3）instead of 不是······而是

Excerpt：

Instead of prescribing treatments that have been developed for the average person，the dream is that we will instead take only treatments that we know will work based on who we are and how we live our lives.

Translation：

_____

_____

（4）set up 建立

Excerpt：

The company has already processed the data of over 300 million patients by setting up cloud services in participating Chinese hospitals or among groups of hospitals.

Translation：

_____

_____

（5）a perfect fit 完美契合；恰到好处

Excerpt：

That's akin to a clothing store only selling suits of three different sizes and expecting a perfect fit for all customers.

Translation：

_____

_____

B. Chinese-English translation

Put the Chinese paragraph into English.

据报道，中国科学家将拟定精准医学计划，以大数据为基础，以基因测序为工具，旨在借助先进的医学技术为特殊疾病和特定患者研究出更具有针对性的诊断和治疗。中国版的精准医学计划将在 4 年内完成 4 000 名志愿者的 DNA 样本和数据的采集。此外，他们将对其中 2 000 人进行精准医学研究，包括全基因组序列分析及以早期预警和干预研究为目的基因组健康分析。精准医学计划对于中国医疗领域及中国社会具有重大意义，因为它不仅能促进一个巨大医疗市场的发展，而且还将有助于提高国家医疗保健的质量和效率。

_____

_____

_____

_____

_____

_____

_____

_____

_____

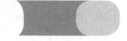
V. Speaking-out Conventional Medicine *vs.* Precision Medicine

1. **Read and say.**

Read the table showing the differences between conventional medicine and precision medicine. Work in pairs to compare and contrast these two medical models.

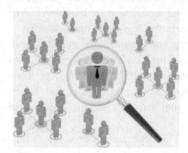

From Disease Care to Health Care
Distinguishing Conventional Medicine from Precision Medicine

	Conventional medicine	Precision medicine
Philosophy	With the exception of an annual "check-up", you visit your doctor when you feel sick.	You visit a precisionist doctor at any time for a precision health analysis that evaluates your current health and anticipates your future health trajectory.
Practice	At the doctor's office, Your symptoms are treated with a textbook, standardized, one-size-fits-all approach.	At the doctor's office, your precision health analysis examines and integrates your metabolomics, hormones, fitness, test results, lifestyle, and genomics, together with detailed family and medical history from complex data to precise direction.
Outcome	You leave the office with instructions to treat the problem that caused your visit.	Your personalized program for lifelong health begins — a collaboration between you and your doctor to detect, predict, and reverse disease at the cellular level.
Goals	You get well.	A healthspan to match your lifespan.

Compare and contrast:

Comparison is an act of examining similarities while contrast is an act of distinguishing by comparing differences. The purpose of comparison and contrast is to analyze the differences and/or the similarities of two distinct subjects. A good comparison/contrast doesn't only point out how the subjects are similar or different (or even both!). It uses those points to make a meaningful argument about the subjects.

There are several ways to organize a comparison-and-contrast structure. Which one you choose depends on what works best for your ideas.

(1) Subject by subject. This organization deals with all of the points about Subject A, then all of the points of Subject B. The strength of this form is that you don't jump back and forth as much between subjects, which can help you speak more smoothly. The major disadvantage is that the comparisons and contrasts don't really become evident, and it can end up speaking like a list of "points" rather than a cohesive speech. Therefore, the following guidelines should be followed to ensure unity:

◇ Each aspect in Subject A must also be discussed in Subject B.

◇ Each aspect should be discussed in the same order in both subjects.

◇ Use appropriate transitional words such as *like/unlike*, *in contrast to*, *compared with* ... and comparative and superlative degrees to achieve unity.

(2) Point by point. This type of organization switches back and forth between points. For example, you could first discuss the prices of frozen pizza *vs.* homemade pizza, then the quality of ingredients, then the convenience factor. The advantage of this form is that it's very clear what you're comparing and contrasting. The disadvantage is that you do switch back and forth between topics, so you need to make sure that you use transitions and signposts to lead your listeners through your argument.

(3) Compare then contrast. This organization presents all the comparisons first, then ends with how your subjects are different (and, usually, how one is superior). It's a pretty common way of organizing a speech, and it works best when you want to emphasize the contrasts between your subjects. Putting the contrasts last places the emphasis on them. However, it can be more difficult for your listeners to immediately see why these two subjects are being contrasted if all the similarities are first.

More useful expressions:

Common transitional words for comparison		Common transitional words for contrast	
similarly	likewise	different from	although
in the same way	besides	in contrast	but
at the same time	also	in spite of	despite
first, second, third, etc.	just as	on the contrary	unlike
equally important	in fact	on the other hand	yet
for one thing	for another	nevertheless	nonetheless
furthermore	moreover	whereas	while
in addition to	then	just the opposite	even though
the same is true of	too	the reverse is true of	

2. **Watch and act**

Watch a video clip. Fill in the blanks and retell the general meaning of the video in class.

Imagine a world where diagnosing an illness is as simple as getting blood drawn, where diseases can be targeted by medicines with (1) _____ , where drugs are perfectly tailored to a patient's genetic makeup and produce no side effects. This world is the promise of precision medicine. And with the growing ease with which (2) _____ can be collected, many believe now may be the best time to start delivering on that promise.

The last decade has witnessed impressive advances in (3) _____ , (4) _____ , (5) _____ and (6) _____. And today more people are engaging in improving their health and participating in health research than ever before.

Dr. Eric Schadt, professor of genomics at the Icahn Institute for Genomics and Multiscale Biology discusses what scientists can do with the universe of data collected from individuals. Capitalizing on the (7) _____ of medical diagnostic technology and the growing popularity of wearable sensors and mobile apps designed for health management. Scientists can aggregate massive amounts of data to create (8) _____ of disease. These models, Dr. Schadt says, can lead to better diagnosis and treatments for common and rare human diseases. The presenters at Precision Medicine 2016 approached the refinement of medical treatments from many angles. From the technical and organizational challenges of (9) _____ of many volunteers, to the computational challenges of accessing and analyzing these vast datasets, to the design challenge of creating treatments that interact with cells and proteins in desirable ways. Together the presenters and participants of Precision Medicine 2016 are paving the way to (10) _____ in medicine and health.

VI. Pros/Cons   Benefited from Precision Medicine

1. Read the following passage with ten statements attached to it. Each statement contains information given in one of the paragraphs. Identify the paragraph from which the information is derived. You may choose a paragraph more than once. Each paragraph is marked with a letter.

_____ (1) Kareem, Six-time NBA Most Valuable Player, recovered from leukemia thanks to precision medicine.

_____ (2) Melanie believed precision medicine offered the hope that her daughter could have additional choices for preserving her health in the future.

119

_____ （3）Targeted therapies were used to treat Steve Jobs' cancer but turned out to be a failure.

_____ （4）The actress Jolie underwent a double mastectomy after having a genetic testing and learning that she might have a higher risk for breast cancer.

_____ （5）Beatrice suffered from a whole new syndrome and her father's team used precision medicine to save her.

_____ （6）Few people can afford Sovaldi although it is the best solution for almost all Hepatitis C patients.

_____ （7）Emily was enrolled in a pioneering cancer immunotherapy trial at the Children's Hospital of Philadelphia.

_____ （8）The database of patients' genetic profiles can lead to inappropriate treatment with bad consequences.

_____ （9）Melanie's family has a history of breast cancer.

_____ （10）Beatrice's father and his team of scientific volunteers spent six years identifying the cause of her condition.

A）Precision medicine is already saving lives. Read the stories of some of the people that have benefited from this new approach.

Emily Whitehead

B） 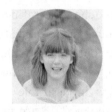 At age six, Emily Whitehead was the first pediatric patient to be treated with a new kind of cancer immunotherapy and was cancer free only 28 days later. "If you didn't know what happened to her, and you saw her now, you would have no idea what she has been through," says Emily's Mom.

C）Her parents decided to enroll her in a pioneering cancer immunotherapy trial at the Children's Hospital of Philadelphia. Emily's T cells were collected from her blood and reengineered in the lab to recognize a protein found only on the surface of leukemia cells. Those T cells were then infused back into Emily's blood, where they circulated throughout her body on a mission to seek and destroy her leukemia. Knowing how to turn these T cells into what Emily called "ninja warriors" required big investments in basic biomedical research. In fact, *Science Magazine* named it a 2013 Breakthrough of the Year — Emily's family couldn't agree more.

Melanie Nix

D） 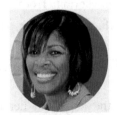 Melanie Nix's family has a history of breast cancer — a history that Melanie couldn't escape when she tested positive for the BRCA gene mutations linked to breast cancer in 2008. After 16 rounds of chemotherapy and breast reconstruction surgery, she had to have both ovaries removed to further reduce risks of cancer in the future. But Melanie is now cancer free thanks to precision medicine.

E) Melanie's positive test results for the BRCA gene mutations instantly concerned her medical team. BRCA gene mutations are linked to breast and ovarian cancers. Further tests confirmed that she had triple-negative breast cancer, a very aggressive form of breast cancer that disproportionately affects African-American women. Her best chance for cancer-free survival was to have a bilateral mastectomy. Melanie says that this type of tailored treatment gave her hope. "Precision medicine offers the hope that by the time my daughter is at an age when she considers genetic testing, new, targeted treatments will be available to give her additional choices for preserving her health," she said.

Hugh and Beatrice Rienhoff

F) 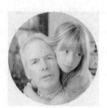 Beatrice Rienhoff's eyes were spaced wider than usual, her leg muscles were weak, and she couldn't gain weight. Her father, a trained clinical geneticist, took notice and wanted to help. After six years, he and his team of scientific volunteers identified the cause of her condition.

G) Beatrice's original medical team had thought her condition resembled Marfan syndrome, a genetic disorder that can cause tears in the human heart. It's typically a fatal syndrome. However, the doctors couldn't fully diagnose Beatrice with Marfan — or any other known disease. Acting as "Super Dad", Hugh lead his team to identifying a variant responsible for his daughter's condition and this research gave rise to the description of a whole new syndrome. The team continues to use precision medicine to learn more about the new syndrome and further study genetic variation to help those like his daughter. Today, Beatrice is living a full life.

Kareem Abdul-Jabbar

H) 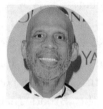 Six-time NBA Most Valuable Player, Kareem Abdul-Jabbar was diagnosed with a form of leukemia in 2008. Known to be lethal, leukemia is a cancer of the blood and bone marrow. It caused the basketball great to slow down, fall ill, and worry. A few years later, he credits precision medicine for helping him to be well today.

Angelina Jolie

I) 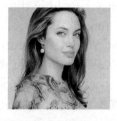 On May 14, 2013, cinema superstar Angelina Jolie announced that she'd had a double mastectomy to prevent the family scourge of breast cancer. With a courageous and medically explicit discussion of her odds and her "medical choice" to remove both breasts, Jolie splashed the issues of cancer prevention and genetic testing for cancer across the front pages.

J) About 10 percent of breast cancers have a genetic component, and two mutations, called BRCA1 and BRCA2, greatly increase the lifetime risk of breast, uterine and other cancers. The BRCA genes normally suppress tumors by repairing broken DNA; when the gene is mutated, both suppression and repair may fail. By itself, the BRCA1 mutation raises the lifetime odds of breast cancer to about 65 percent, about five times the US average. The odds are higher if, as in Jolie's case, many relatives have the cancer.

K) Enthusiasm for precision medicine, from the White House down to everyday physicians, is at an all-time high. But there exist some serious problems and failure cases.

Inappropriate Treatment

L) The databases used to interpret patients' genetic profiles can lead to "inappropriate treatment" with "devastating consequences", researchers at the Mayo Clinic once warned. Their report describes the cases of some two dozen people who were told they had a potentially fatal illness and one who had a heart defibrillator surgically implanted but, it turns out, never needed it. The individuals were family members who underwent genetic testing after a young relative died of a heart syndrome. Test results indicated that they carried a mutation in a heart-related gene — and the database that the testing company used indicated it caused a serious disorder.

A Dilemma at Every Income Level

M) This dilemma applies to more than the poor and downtrodden. Many people in the US at every income level below the top 1% find themselves in untenable circumstances affecting their health. Take for example, the new Hepatitis C drug, Sovaldi, which cures almost all patients of the disease. Precision medicine and big data analysis will inevitably point to Sovaldi as the best solution for almost all Hepatitis C patients. After all, it is the only known cure for a previously incurable, potentially lethal disease. But the makers of that drug, Gilead Sciences, attached an $84,000 price tag to the drug. Few can afford that. Even insurance companies can't afford it. The upshot is that access and affordability of many treatments is a problem for the vast majority of patients no matter their income level or insurance plan.

Steve Jobs

N) 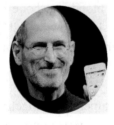 Walter Isaacson's biography of Steve Jobs revealed that after his cancer had recurred as metastatic disease in 2010, Jobs had consulted with research teams at Stanford, Johns Hopkins, and the Broad Institute to have the genome of his cancer and normal tissue sequenced, one of the first twenty people in the world to have this information. At the time (2010 – 2011), each genome sequence cost $100,000, which Jobs could easily afford. Scientists and oncologists looked at this information and used it to choose various targeted therapies for Jobs throughout the remainder of his life, and Jobs met with all his doctors and researchers from the three institutions working on the DNA from his cancer at the Four Seasons Hotel in Palo Alto to discuss the genetic signatures found in Jobs' cancer and how best to target them. Jobs' case, as we now know, was a failure. However much Jobs' team tried to stay one step ahead of his cancer, the cancer caught up and passed whatever they could do.

2. Read the following statements. Decide to what extent you agree or disagree with each statement, and write your own pros or cons in the box, then set out your rational viewpoints and the reasons.

(1) Precision medicine is superior to conventional medicine.
(2) Diagnosis can be improved through precision medicine.
(3) Each patient can benefit from precision medicine.

Pros	Cons

VII. Outcome Sentence Analysis and Essay Writing

1. Sentence-structure analysis

Aanalyze the following sentences and draw a tree-structure.

(1) For example, even if someone inherits genetic variations that make them susceptible to skin cancer, they can decrease their chances of getting cancer by protecting themselves from the sun.

(2) Progressing even farther, a team of researchers recently announced the development of a prototype computer algorithm that can print 3D drugs with personalized information.

（3）Instead of prescribing treatments that have been developed for the average person，the dream is that we will instead take only treatments that we know will work based on who we are and how we live our lives.

2. **Essay writing**

   Write an essay on the precision medicine. Search for relevant information via the Internet or books in the library. The following outline is for your reference.

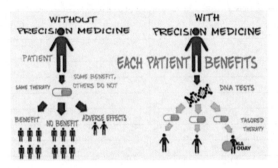

   Outline：

   （1）What is precision medicine? What's the current situation of precision medicine?

   （2）Benefits of precision medicine.

   （3）Controversies of precision medicine.

   （4）Your views on precision medicine.

   _____
   _____
   _____
   _____
   _____
   _____
   _____
   _____
   _____
   _____
   _____
   _____

Unit 5
Big Data Medicine

Read the web page. Then answer the questions orally.

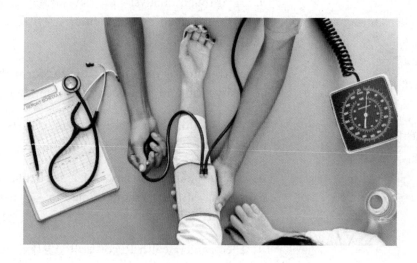

Big data in healthcare is a term used to describe massive volumes of information created by the adoption of digital technologies that collect patients' records and help in managing hospital performance, otherwise too large and complex for traditional technologies.

The application of big data analytics in healthcare has a lot of positive and also lifesaving outcomes. In essence, big-style data refers to the vast quantities of information created by the digitization of everything, that gets consolidated and analyzed by specific technologies. Applied to healthcare, it will use specific health data of a population (or of a particular individual) and potentially help to prevent epidemics, cure disease, cut down costs, etc.

That said, the amount of sources in which health professionals can gain insights

125

from their patients keeps growing. This data is normally coming in different formats and sizes，which presents a challenge to the user. However，the current focus is no longer on how "big" the data is，but on how smartly is managed. With the help of the right technology，data can be extracted from the following sources of the big data in healthcare industry in a smart and fast way：

- Patients portals
- Research studies
- EHRs
- Wearable devices
- Search engines
- Generic databases
- Government agencies
- Payer records
- Staffing schedules
- Patient waiting room

analytics [ˌænəˈlɪtɪks]	*n*. a through analysis of data using a model，usually performed by a computer（通常通过计算机利用模型所做的）数据分析
digitization [ˌdɪdʒɪtaɪˈzeɪʃən]	*n*. conversion of data into a digital form that can be easily read and processed by a computer 数字化
consolidate [kənˈsɒlɪdeɪt]	*v*. to join things together into one；to be joined into one（使）结成一体，合并
epidemic [ˌepɪˈdemɪk]	*n*. a large number of cases of a particular disease happening at the same time in a particular community 流行病
EHRs	*n*. Electronic Health Records 电子健康记录

(1) What does big data refer to in healthcare?

_____

(2) What is the application of big data analytics?

_____

(3) What is the current focus for big data medicine?

_____

II. Watching-in Big Data in Healthcare

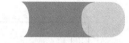

1. **View the video clips. Match the photos (A – D) to the dialogues (1 – 4). Then answer the following questions.**

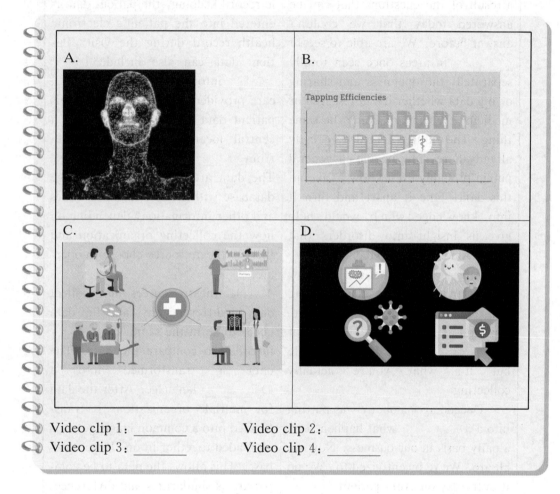

A.

B.
Tapping Efficiencies

C.

D.

Video clip 1: _____   Video clip 2: _____

Video clip 3: _____   Video clip 4: _____

(1) What technology can be applied to collect data according to video 1?

_____

(2) What do researchers mean when they use the term "big data" according to video 2?

_____

(3) What is the goal of healthcare analytics according to video 3?

_____

(4) Why systematic analysis of extensive data is more effective according to video 4?

_____

2. View the video clips again. Fill in the blanks to complete the sentences which can help you get the gist of the content.

(1)

This is the most exciting time in my entire career, and I think that is a result of the questions that can be answered today that we couldn't answer before. We are able to see 1) _____ in areas once seen totally separated, the openness and sharing of big data whether it's in research or medicine. It's sort of doing the same thing. The future of health is really already here, few people in general public probably even know. Take all this data, take it apart and turn it into knowledge which would help give us insight into disorders that affect Americans everyday.

And it's the notion of now putting that into data elements and data elements that we can search. Big data is not just the number of 2) _____ that are in your sample but it's what you're actually collecting.

Decade ago, nobody was putting into a 3) _____ what happened on a daily basis in our business. Now we all are. We're incentivized to. We do it every day on every patient.

(2)

When a patient visits a healthcare office or clinic that has electronic record-keeping, the patient data is entered into the patient's electronic health record during the visit. Patient data can also include 1) _____ information like the health care providers notes. A copy of this patient data is then sent over to a central location that collects data from 2) _____ healthcare sources. The data are collected into a large database with notes, diagnosis codes and other information, depending on how the collecting organization and the healthcare source choose to operate.

Healthcare sources may collect data in different ways and the data needs to be in the same 3) _____ in order to compare the data. The data is transformed into a 4) _____ language. After the data for multiple organizations is transformed into a common language, it is all loaded together in one large database. This allows the data to be compared, as similarities and differences are now easier to 5) _____ because the data is in the same format. Researchers then receive the data to use in a research study. This is typically done by submitting a question to the collecting organization to see if a

<table>
<tr>
<td></td>
<td>population of interest exists before attempting a research study. This is called the cohort discovery.</td>
</tr>
<tr>
<td>

(3)

What do you think happened to all that medical data about you? Does your current doctor have 1) _____ to it? Most of our medical history depends on what we remember to write down on that form when we first show up, which isn't very reliable. And I'm not sure anyone even looks at those. This is where analytics can 2) _____ healthcare and there are a lot of cool companies working on this. But there are some big challenges for data professionals to tackle. There are a number of goals that the healthcare industry hopes analytics can help with, potentially helping to prevent epidemics, cure elusive diseases, reduce costs and improve quality of life. By collecting large amounts of data from the population, 3) _____ analytics can help detect and prevent serious illness before it happens. Getting treatments before patients may even be showing signs.
</td>
<td>

(4)

Today's vast amount of medical data needs to be integrated and accessed intelligently to support better healthcare 1) _____. Big data made smart can create new networks of knowledge sharing. By measuring and monitoring processes 2) _____, we can compare data more easily. Such insights facilitate streamlined workflows, greater efficiencies, and improved patient care. Systematic analysis of extensive data can help to detect patterns so that clinicians can tailor treatment to individuals and project health outcomes. Digital networks can bring together partners and knowledge sharing. Delivering context relevant clinical information at the point of care enables more holistic 3) _____. Healthcare can only benefit from big data when it is made structured, relevant, smart and accessible.
</td>
</tr>
</table>

| incentivize [ɪnˈsentɪvaɪz] | v. to encourage sb to do sth, especially by offering them a reward 激励,鼓励 |
| cohort [ˈkəʊhɔːt] | n. a group of people who share a common feature or aspect of behaviour（有共同特点或举止类同的）一群人,一批人 |

streamline ['striːmlaɪn]	*v.* to make a system, an organization, etc. work better, especially in a way that saves money 使(系统、机构等)效率更高;(尤指)使增产节约
holistic [həʊ'lɪstɪk]	
workflow ['wɜːkfləʊ]	*n.* progress (or rate of progress) in work being done 工作流程
holistic [həʊ'lɪstɪk]	*adj.* treating the whole person rather than just the symptoms (=effects) of a disease 功能整体性的

III. Leading-in Defining Big Data

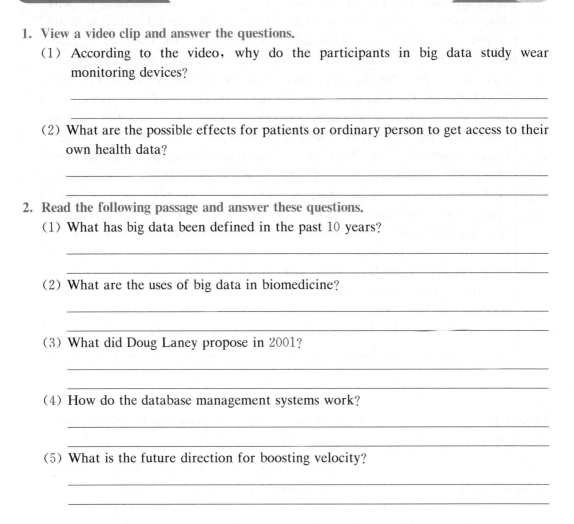

1. **View a video clip and answer the questions.**
   (1) According to the video, why do the participants in big data study wear monitoring devices?
   _____

   (2) What are the possible effects for patients or ordinary person to get access to their own health data?
   _____
   _____

2. **Read the following passage and answer these questions.**
   (1) What has big data been defined in the past 10 years?
   _____

   (2) What are the uses of big data in biomedicine?
   _____

   (3) What did Doug Laney propose in 2001?
   _____

   (4) How do the database management systems work?
   _____

   (5) What is the future direction for boosting velocity?
   _____
   _____

Passage A

Big Health Data: What Are They?

In the last decade, "big data" has been used to define a research approach involving the use of large-scale, complex datasets. Although difficult, it may be defined as a "cultural, technological, and scholarly phenomenon" based on the application of machine learning algorithms to data process and analysis. In biomedical research, big data is used for electronic health record (EHR) considered "relevant" to the understanding of health and disease, including clinical, imaging, omic, data from internet use and wearable devices, and others. The basic principle is to make the whole biomedical practice "evidence generating" without the need to design and conduct ad hoc studies. The most popular description for big data was proposed by Doug Laney in 2001 and is known in the academic world as the "3Vs": volume, variety, and velocity.

Volume

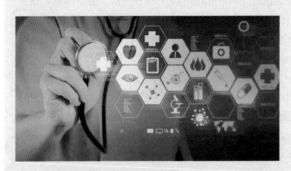

An unimaginable amount of data is created every year and only a very small part is used for research. Since the total amount of data is projected to double every 2 years, in 2020 we are having 50 times more data (44 zettabytes, or 44 trillion gigabytes) than in 2011. To give an idea, 1 kilobyte is the size of a page of text, 1 gigabyte correspond to about 6 millions of books, and a typical large tertiary care hospital generates about 100 terabytes of data per year. This explosion lies in the possibility to store huge quantity of data, as the average price of gigabyte of storage fell in the last 30 years, and easy access to them.

High sample size is required to investigate both rare and common CVD (particularly if the endpoint is infrequent). From the end of the Second World War to today, the volume of logs (first in the United States, then in Europe) has been gradually increasing. The Framingham study started in 1948 and enrolled 5,209 patients in its original cohort. Subsequently, the population increased with additional cohorts (offspring, third generation, new offspring spouse, Omni 1 and Omni 2) and to date counts more than 15 thousands subjects. In 2014, through a nationwide enrollment of patients with ischemic heart disease, the SWEDEHEART registry included 105,674 patients with ST-elevation myocardial infarction (STEMI) and 205,693 with non-ST-elevation myocardial infarction (NSTEMI).

Variety

Historically，the majority of EHR were structured in spreadsheet or databases. However，the variety of data has become much less congruent and stored in countless forms with a growing trend toward "unstructured" format. Structured data are highly-organized informations easy to 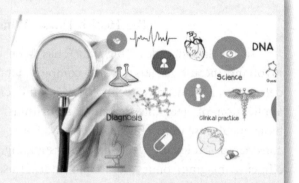 process and analyze. Examples of structured CVD data are：age，drug doses，lab values，electrocardiogram（ECG），echocardiographic values，genetic data（e. g. single nucleotide polymorphisms，copy number variations and rare mutations），tools for genetic analysis（e. g. arrays and next-generation sequencing），etc. Unstructured data do not have a predefined data model or schema，and may be textual or nontextual，human- or machine-generated. However，many unstructured informations may be helpful to assemble a holistic view of a patient，including social and environmental factors potentially influencing health. Among them we can find：medical instructions，differential diagnosis，reports，digital clinical notes，physical examination，but also blogs，tweets，and Facebook posting. Most of the database management systems through interchange and translation mechanism allow us to overcome the barriers of the past related to the variety of incompatible data formats，nonaligned data，and inconsistent data semantics. The technical obstacles in linking such variety of informations is one of the main challenge of big data analytics. For example，the absence of a unique patient identifier in the United States has limited the linkage of data for research purpose. However，the development of increasingly sophisticated probabilistic algorithms based on the available demographics data（e. g. name，age，zip code，etc.）allows linking informations with an acceptable risk of error.

Velocity

Big data must provide solutions that reduce the time for storing and retrieving of data packets (so called "data latency"). Velocity，in fact，requires architectures which do not assume that the informations must be near real time. The enterprises have developed solution such as operational data stores which periodically extract and reorganize data for operational inquiry，caches providing instant access to the informations，and point-to-point data routing between apps and databases. Another possible future direction to boost velocity is the application of "anytime algorithms" that can learn from streaming data and that return a valuable result if their execution is stopped at any time.

volume [ˈvɒljuːm]	*n*. the amount of 3-dimensional space occupied by an object 体积, 容积; 总数, 总量
velocity [vɪˈlɒsətɪ]	*n*. a high speed 高速
kilobyte [ˈkɪləbaɪt]	*n*. a unit of information equal to 1 024 bytes [计] 千字节, 1 024 字节
congruent [ˈkɒŋgruənt]	*adj*. having the same size and shape; fitting together well 全等的; 一致的, 适合的
mutation [mjuːˈteɪʃən]	*n*. the act or process of being altered or changed 变异
probabilistic [ˌprɒbəbɪˈlɪstɪk]	*adj*. (of methods, arguments, etc.) based on the idea that, as we cannot be certain about things, we can base our beliefs or actions on what is probable 概率性的; 盖然论的
latency [ˈleɪtənsɪ]	*n*. the time that elapses between a stimulus and the response to it 延迟

Unit 1　Unit 2　Unit 3　Unit 4　Unit 5　Unit 6　Unit 7　Unit 8

3. **Match each of the terms listed below with the numbered definition. Write the letter in the space provided.**

A. wearable	B. schema	C. ischemic
D. analytics	E. spreadsheet	F. specialist
G. periodically	H. latency	I. unstructured
J. inquiry	K. velocity	L. accumulated

(1) _____ : lacking definite structure or organization

(2) _____ : the discovery and communication of meaningful patterns in data

(3) _____ : high speed

(4) _____ : an instance of questioning

(5) _____ : an internal representation of the world; an organization of concepts and actions that can be revised by new information about the world

(6) _____ : brought together into a group or crowd

(7) _____ : a covering designed to be worn on a person's body

(8) _____ : the time that elapses between a stimulus and the response to it

(9) _____ : a screen-oriented interactive program enabling a user to lay out financial data on the screen

(10) _____ : an expert who is devoted to one occupation or branch of learning

(11) _____ : relating to or affected by ischemia

(12) _____ : in a sporadic manner

IV. Critical Reading | Further Reading on Big Data in Medicine

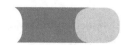

1. Big Data in Medicine, the Present and Hopefully the Future

Read the following passage and fill in the blanks to complete the table.

Issues	Descriptions
Health	It represents a "state of complete (1) _____, mental, and social well-being, and not merely the absence of disease or (2) _____".
Antibiotics	The introduction of antibiotics, but also the ability to treat a vast array of (3) _____ have improved not only (4) _____ _____, but also the quality of life.
Biological data	They have not provided (5) _____ to discern the feature of individuals within populations, nor to cater reliable predictive markers, and yet there is a widespread (6) _____, that their (7) _____ would (8) _____ improve the management of patients and more broadly of the individual health status.
Smart phones and portable devices	Applications is promising a more (9) _____, robust mean to record, organize and (10) _____ the various information included in this realm.
Nonnegative Matrix Factorization	NMF and more recently (11) _____ have gained traction, and appear to provide at last (12) _____ toward this goal. NMF was first proposed as a method to (13) _____
Multi-Omics Factor Analysis	It aims to infer hidden factors underlying biological and technical sources of (14) _____. To this end, MOFA defines axes of (15) _____, either shared or specific across (16) _____ _____.
EU General Data Protection Regulation	GDPR is a (17) _____ attempt to protect (18) _____ of the individuals, while fostering research and more specifically free scientific (19) _____.
Clinicians	They would have to engage and interact more (20) _____ with clinical laboratory technicians and researchers to work more closely together.

Big Data in Medicine, the Present and Hopefully the Future

Introduction

As stated by the World Health Organization (WHO), health represents a "state of complete physical, mental, and social well-being, and not merely the absence of disease or infirmity". The introduction of antibiotics, but also the ability to treat a vast array of ailments have improved not only life expectancy, but also the quality of life. We are now entering another era, which will be centered upon big data and that has been heralded, possibly with some exaggeration, revolutionary. We posit that this new perspective is endowed with unique opportunities, but also with menacing threats, which need to be promptly addressed, provided also the unparalleled intrusive capacity of new technologies.

Beyond the Genome

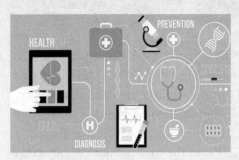

Beside the collection and the analysis of biological data, other data sets are entering the arena of personalized medicine. Up to this point, they have not provided robust metrics to discern the feature of individuals within populations, nor to cater reliable predictive markers, and yet there is a widespread enthusiasm and thrust, that their implementation would significantly improve the management of patients and more broadly of the individual health status. A case in point is represented by the exposome, whose goal is to collect a vast array of data, deemed crucial for the well-being, which include diet, pollution, and stress, among others. While the collection of these data may appear (and still is) ephemeral, the introduction of new technologies, including applications in smartphones and portable devices, is promising a more standardized, robust mean to record, organize and track the various information included in this realm.

Challenges of Data Integration

Nonnegative Matrix Factorization (NMF) and more recently Multi-Omics Factor Analysis (MOFA) have gained traction, and appear to provide at last inroads toward this goal. NMF was first proposed as a method to decompose images, for example, faces into parts reminiscent of features such as eyes, nose, mouth, cheeks, and chin. It has been then applied to microarray data, where it was able to reduce the dimension of expression data from thousands of genes to a few metagenes. We then applied NMF for the first time to the analysis of DNA copy number variation data. Lately, NMF has been used to integrate data from different sources, e.g. single cell RNA and single cell ATAC-seq data. Another promising tool to integrate data is MOFA，which aims to infer hidden factors underlying biological and technical sources of variability. To this end，MOFA defines axes of heterogeneity，either shared or specific across data modalities.

Ethical Challenges，the GDPR，and Beyond

The availability of "big data" is posing significant challenges also from an ethical standpoint. The recent introduction in the European community of the EU General Data Protection Regulation（GDPR）is a comprehensive attempt to protect privacy rights of the individuals，while fostering research and more specifically free scientific data exchange. Despite its considerable

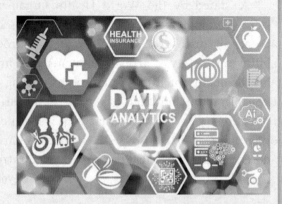

sanctionatory harshness（up to 4% of a company's yearly global revenues，in case of noncompliance），the general philosophy underlying the GDPR revolves around decentralization，through the delegation of responsibility to data controllers. Additionally，the GDPR increases the role of internal review boards（IRBs）and ethical committees，with an enhanced role in policy making. Albeit it is too early to properly assess the impact and the role of GDPR in the management of big data，nevertheless it is certain that tensions will arise around the management of the data and to properly regulate their use and who could assess them.

The Future：Participatory Medicine

As noted above，the new era of big data in medicine provides several new challenges，alongside great opportunities，to improve the health for human kind，not only for wealthy nations，but also for underdeveloped countries. To this end，it is fair to say that a profound cultural shift ought to occur，which entails professional figures and stakeholders that up to now have not been engaged in previous revolutions. Patients，doctors，but also clinical laboratory technicians and researchers would need to acquire new knowledge，and most relevantly interact and acquire novel frames of mind and perspectives，leading to an entirely overhauled health ecosystem. Clinicians would have to engage and interact more pervasively with clinical laboratory technicians and researchers to work more closely together.

We hope that this goal is not overambitious and could be reached in a future not too far.

infirmity [ɪnˈfɜːmətɪ]	*n*. the state of being weak in health or body (especially from old age) (尤指老年的)体弱，病弱
herald [ˈherəld]	*v*. to say in public that sb/sth is good or important 宣称(……是好的或重要的)
endow [ɪnˈdaʊ]	*v*. give qualities or abilities to 给予；赋予
reminiscent [ˌremɪˈnɪsənt]	*adj*. serving to bring to mind 使人联想的；与……相像的
heterogeneity [ˌhetərəʊdʒɪˈniːətɪ]	*n*. the quality of being diverse and not comparable in kind 异质性；非均匀性
stakeholder [ˈsteɪkˌhəʊldə(r)]	*n*. a person or company that is involved in a particular organization, project, system, etc., especially because they have invested money in it (某组织、工程、体系等的)参与人；有权益关系者
pervasively [pɜːˈveɪsɪvlɪ]	*adv*. existing in all parts of a place or thing 遍布地；普遍地

2. **Unleashing the Power of Big Data to Guide Precision Medicine in China**

Read the following passage to complete the note-taking table, and then check your understanding.

Year	Event
2004	(1) _____, a chronic-disease initiative was launched. It recruited more than (2) _____ adults from 10 regions across China in its first 4 years, collecting data through (3) _____.
2016	Precision medicine in China was given a boost when the government included the field in its (4) _____ economic plan. (5) _____ is part of the Healthy China 2030 plan, also launched this year.
2016 – 2018	MOST has invested about (6) _____ in more than 100 projects. These range from finding new drug targets for (7) _____.
2017 – 2019	Li Fei led a phase Ⅱ clinical trial of (8) _____ as a potential treatment for life-altering symptoms in children with (9) _____.
2019	The Chinese government set up two open-access data centers to encourage (10) _____ — the National Genomics Data Center and its umbrella organization, the China National Center for Bioinformation — but not every research project (11) _____ its data.
2021	Another (12) _____ project launched, after Yuan Huijun, a physician who has been researching hereditary hearing loss for more than (13) _____.
2025	The institute plans to set up a database of 100,000 people from China who have (14) _____, including spinal muscular (15) _____ and albinism.

Passage C

Unleashing the Power of Big Data to Guide Precision Medicine in China

Between 2017 and 2019, Li Fei led a phase II clinical trial of the drug bumetanide as a potential treatment for life-altering symptoms in children with autism spectrum disorder (ASD). Li, a developmental-behavioural paediatrician at Xinhua Hospital in Shanghai, China, saw that in some children, the drug reduced the severity of ASD symptoms such as profound difficulties with communication. But in others, it had no effect at all.

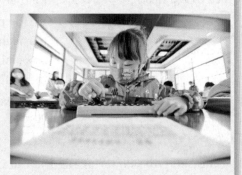

Many medical therapies use a "one-size-fits-all" strategy. But because of individual variability in genes, environments and lifestyles, people with the same condition might not respond to a single treatment in the same way. To understand these variations, scientists worldwide are tapping into large data sets, hoping to identify molecular patterns for particular conditions. Together with genetic testing, that would allow clinicians to select treatments that are tailored to individuals — an approach known as precision medicine.

Heavy Investment

Precision medicine in China was given a boost in 2016 when the government included the field in its 13th five-year economic plan. The policy blueprint, which defined the country's spending priorities until 2020, pledged to "spur innovation and industrial application" in precision medicine alongside other areas such as smart vehicles and new materials.

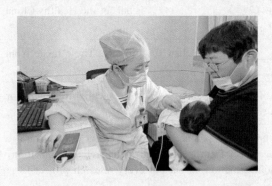

Precision medicine is part of the Healthy China 2030 plan, also launched in 2016. The idea is to use the approach to tackle some major healthcare challenges the country faces, such as rising cancer rates and issues related to an aging population. Current projections suggest that, by 2040, 28% of China's population will be over 60 years old.

Following the announcement of the five-year plan, China's Ministry of Science and Technology (MOST) launched a precision-medicine project as part of its National Key Research and Development Program. MOST has invested about 1. 3 billion *yuan* (US $ 200. 4 million) in more than 100 projects from 2016 to 2018.

These range from finding new drug targets for chronic diseases such as diabetes to developing better sequencing technologies and building a dozen large population cohorts comprising hundreds of thousands of people from across China.

China's population of 1. 4 billion people means the country has great potential for using big data to study health issues, says Chen Zhengming, an epidemiologist and chronic-disease researcher at the University of Oxford, UK. "The advantage is especially prominent in the research of rare diseases, where you might not be able to have a data set in smaller countries like the United Kingdom, where only a handful of cases exist," says Chen, who leads the China Kadoorie Biobank, a chronic-disease initiative that launched in 2004. It recruited more than 510,000 adults from 10 regions across China in its first 4 years, collecting data through questionnaires and by recording physical measurements and storing participants' blood samples for future study.

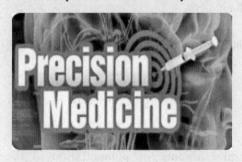

Another big-data precision-medicine project launched in 2021, after Yuan Huijun, a physician who has been researching hereditary hearing loss for more than two decades, founded the Institute of Rare Diseases at West China Hospital in Chengdu, Sichuan Province, in 2020. By 2025, the institute plans to set up a database of 100,000 people from China who have rare conditions, including spinal muscular atrophy and albinism. It will contain basic health information and data relating to biological samples, such as blood for gene sequencing. Rare diseases are hard to diagnose, because their incidences are low.

Challenges Ahead

As the funding cycle for many of the precision-medicine projects financed since 2016 ends, ongoing support will become crucial, says Chen — particularly given that cohorts usually take several years to build and are time-consuming and costly to maintain.

Financial support from MOST's precision-medicine programme is usually for 4 – 5 years, and the amount — less than 20 million *yuan* per cohort study — is far from enough to sequence the genomes of the tens of thousands of participants enrolled in them. Using MOST's funding, many of these large cohorts have just started in the past few years.

Data sharing presents an additional challenge, in part because China's health data are fragmented across various repositories, research teams and hospitals. In 2019, the Chinese government set up two open-access data centers to encourage data sharing — the National Genomics Data Center and its umbrella organization, the China National Center for Bioinformation — but not every research project deposits its data.

"We invested so much in building such a big platform, and we're hoping to share it with other teams across the country. After we bring these fragmented resources together, the data will generate more value. It's a win-win situation," Yuan concludes.

paediatrician [ˌpiːdɪəˈtrɪʃən]	*n.* a specialist in the care of babies 儿科医生;儿科学家
severity [sɪˈverətɪ]	*n.* the fact or condition of sth being extremely bad or serious 严重;严重性
spinal [ˈspaɪnəl]	*adj.* of or relating to the spine or spinal cord 脊髓的;脊柱的
atrophy [ˈætrəfɪ]	*n.* a decrease in size of an organ caused by disease or disuse 萎缩
albinism [ˈælbɪnɪzəm]	*n.* the congenital absence of pigmentation in the eyes, skin and hair 白化病;白化型

3. **Lexical chunks and sentence rewriting**

A. **Substitute the underlined part with the words or expressions you have learned.**

(1) Although difficult, it may <u>be regarded as</u> a "cultural, technological, and scholarly phenomenon" based on the application of machine learning algorithms to data process and analysis. (passage A)

Answer:

Although difficult, it may _____ a "cultural, technological, and scholarly phenomenon" based on the application of machine learning algorithms to data process and analysis.

(2) The Framingham study started in 1948 and <u>entered</u> 5,209 patients in its original cohort. (passage A)

Answer:

The Framingham study started in 1948 and _____ 5,209 patients in its original cohort.

(3) As <u>declared</u> by the World Health Organization (WHO), health represents a "state of complete physical, mental, and social well-being, and not merely the absence of disease or infirmity". (passage B)

Answer:

As _____ by the World Health Organization（WHO）, health represents a "state of complete physical, mental, and social well-being, and not merely the absence of disease or infirmity".

(4) We are now entering another era, which will <u>be focus on</u> big data and that has been heralded, possibly with some exaggeration, revolutionary.（passage B）

Answer:

We are now entering in another era, which will _____ big data and that has been heralded, possibly with some exaggeration, revolutionary.

(5) We posit that this new perspective <u>is borne with</u> unique opportunities, but also with menacing threats, which need to be promptly addressed, provided also the unparalleled intrusive capacity of new technologies.（passage B）

Answer:

We posit that this new perspective _____ unique opportunities, but also with menacing threats, which need to be promptly addressed, provided also the unparalleled intrusive capacity of new technologies.

(6) <u>Sooner or later</u>, they have not provided robust metrics to discern the feature of individuals within populations, nor to cater reliable predictive markers, and yet there is a widespread enthusiasm and thrust.（passage B）

Answer:

_____, they have not provided robust metrics to discern the feature of individuals within populations, nor to cater reliable predictive markers, and yet there is a widespread enthusiasm and thrust.

(7) Despite its considerable sanctionatory harshness, the general philosophy underlying the GDPR <u>centers upon</u> decentralization, through the delegation of responsibility to data controllers.（passage B）

Answer:

Despite its considerable sanctionatory harshness, the general philosophy underlying the GDPR _____ decentralization, through the delegation of responsibility to data controllers.

(8) But in others, it <u>had no influence</u> at all.（passage C）

Answer:

But in others, it _____ at all.

(9) To understand these variations, scientists worldwide <u>are using</u> large data sets, hoping to identify molecular patterns for particular conditions.（passage C）

Answer:

To understand these variations, scientists worldwide _____ large data sets, hoping to identify molecular patterns for particular conditions.

(10) The policy blueprint, which defined the country's spending priorities until 2020, <u>swore to</u> "spur innovation and industrial application" in precision medicine alongside other areas such as smart vehicles and new materials.（passage C）

Answer：

The policy blueprint，which defined the country's spending priorities until 2020，_____ "spur innovation and industrial application" in precision medicine alongside other areas such as smart vehicles and new materials.

B. Rewrite the following sentences using the academic expressions you have learned in the articles.

(1) But in others，it had no influence at all.

Lexical chunks：_____

Sentence rewriting：_____

_____

(2) The Framingham study started in 1948 and entered 5,209 patients in its original cohort.

Lexical chunks：_____

Sentence rewriting：_____

_____

(3) Despite its considerable sanctionatory harshness，the general philosophy underlying the GDPR centers upon decentralization，through the delegation of responsibility to data controllers.

Lexical chunks：_____

Sentence rewriting：_____

_____

(4) To understand these variations，scientists worldwide are using large data sets，hoping to identify molecular patterns for particular conditions.

Lexical chunks：_____

Sentence rewriting：_____

_____

(5) The policy blueprint，which defined the country's spending priorities until 2020，swore to "spur innovation and industrial application" in precision medicine alongside other areas such as smart vehicles and new materials.

Lexical chunks：_____

Sentence rewriting：_____

_____

4. **Bilingual translation**

Put the following into Chinese or vice versa.

A. **English-Chinese translation**

Learn the following useful expressions by translating the sentences selected from the passages.

(1) be defined as 被定义为……

Excerpt：

Although difficult，it may be defined as a "cultural，technological，and scholarly phenomenon" based on the application of machine learning algorithms to data process and analysis.

Translation:

_____

_____

(2) be endowed with 被赋予；天生具有

Excerpt:

We posit that this new perspective is endowed with unique opportunities, but also with menacing threats, which need to be promptly addressed, provided also the unparalleled intrusive capacity of new technologies.

Translation:

_____

_____

(3) revolve around 围绕……转动；以……为中心

Excerpt:

Despite its considerable sanctionatory harshness, the general philosophy underlying the GDPR revolves around decentralization, through the delegation of responsibility to data controllers.

Translation:

_____

_____

(4) enroll 登记；使加入；把……记入名册

Excerpt:

The Framingham study started in 1948 and enrolled 5,209 patients in its original cohort.

Translation:

_____

_____

(5) tap into 利用，发掘（已有的资源、知识等）

Excerpt:

To understand these variations, scientists worldwide are tapping into large data sets, hoping to identify molecular patterns for particular conditions.

Translation:

_____

_____

B. Chinese-English translation

Put the Chinese paragraph into English.

中国将重点促进大数据在医学上的应用。2016 年 6 月，中国国务院就医疗保健行业大数据的发展和使用情况发布了正式通知。国务院认为，卫生和医学领域的大数据是一种国家战略资源，它们的发展可以改善中国的医疗保健。国务院制定了相应的规划发展目标、关键任务和组织框架。继在上海和宁波建立区域卫生数据中心后，国家卫生和计划生育委员会在 2016 年宣布，中国将建立更多的区域性和国家性中心和工业园区，其重点在于将卫生和医学数据作为国家试点项目的一部分，并充分利用这些数据发挥作用。我们选择了中国东部省份福建和江苏的 4 个城市作为试点地点，这些中心目前正在建设中。

_____
_____
_____
_____
_____
_____
_____
_____
_____
_____

V. Speaking-out   Perception About China's Big Data in Healthcare

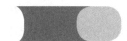

1. Read and say

Part 1: China is committed to applying big data in healthcare programs. How do you value China's endeavor in this field and what they have achieved so far? What difficulties or obstacles do you think China might encounter in gathering people's healthcare data?

Part 2: Please acquire further information of big data's development of healthcare in China. What do you think are the major challenges for big data healthcare to develop in China? What is the future of big data in medicine in China, and how it can be better promoted?

Part 1: What Data Are Gathered in China and How?

China is already making use of big data. The country's personal identification system could be used to link data from various sources. Medical claims data from the national social insurance system have been used to generate a 5% sampling database and an overall database covering over 0.6 billion beneficiaries in the past five years, which are available to scientific researchers. Applications to use these data are managed by organisations such as the Chinese Health Insurance Research Association; there is no public access.

Since 2016, many academic research projects using these national data sets have been approved to evaluate the current and future clinical and economic burden of chronic diseases such as cardiovascular disease, diabetes, kidney disease, and chronic obstructive pulmonary disease. Furthermore, other national administrative databases, including the national standardized discharge summary of inpatients and the national death registry, with hundreds of millions of patient records, have been used by medical and public health researchers.

China is also focusing on personalizing medicine. Since 2016, the Ministry of Science and Technology has initiated and funded many "precision medicine" projects under the national key research and development programme. A centralized and integrated data platform for precision medicine is being developed, which will store all patient/population data as well as biosamples collected from a series of large cohort studies and from biobanks. The platform is expected to include at least 0.7 million participants, 0.4 million from the general population and 0.3 million from patients with major noncommunicable diseases. China's large population base and centralized governance mean that very large sample sizes can be reached, which is of great value to personalized medicine initiatives.

As well as the government-led projects, Chinese academic medical societies are leading data-sharing initiatives. In October 2017, the School of Public Health at Peking University announced the launch of the China Cohort Consortium (chinacohort.bjmu.edu.cn/home). Currently 20 cohorts with more than 2 million participants are included. The activities of the consortium include using common data models for data harmonization, performing individual participant data meta-analyses, and generating new cohorts. Furthermore, disease-based data sharing platforms, including for cardiovascular disease, stroke, cancer, and kidney disease, have been established by medical specialists with the support of the government. For example, the China Kidney Disease Network, which launched in 2015, integrates various sources of data on kidney disease and uses new analytic techniques to provide evidence for healthcare policy, strengthen academic research, and promote effective disease management.

Part 2: Opportunities to Improve Health

The use of big data in medicine includes public health promotion (disease monitoring and population management), healthcare management (quality control and performance measurement), drug and medical device surveillance, routine clinical practice (risk prediction, diagnosis accuracy, and decision support), and research.

The existing mandatory national administrative databases in China produce big data that can easily be used to monitor trends in major diseases and provide evidence for policymaking in healthcare. New data analytics, such as machine learning, to replace much of the work of radiologists and anatomical pathologists, can also be used and is an active area of research in China. However, for applications that need detailed and high-quality clinical information and long term follow-up, such as predicting long term outcomes and providing support for clinical decisions, the data systems in China need to be developed further.

In China, discussion on big data in medicine has focused on how to collect, store, integrate, and manage data and has been led by computer scientists, and the health information industry. However, the future of big data in medicine is in using new analytic techniques such as machine learning to answer clinical questions, educating doctors and policymakers to understand big data, and promoting the use of tools generated by big data and big data technologies that support clinical decision making.

2. Watch and act

Watch a video clip. Fill in the blanks and retell the general meaning of the video in class.

Artificial intelligence is (1) _____ medicine, but how can this (2) _____ be used in the best possible way? For example, if a patient is worried about their health, they can quickly obtain (3) _____ diagnoses with a symptom check app. The app also helps patients decide whether they should see a (4) _____. And if so, which one? The acts of algorithms provides the doctor with (5) _____ information for taking the patient's medical history, even in the case of rare diseases and it can support the choice of the right treatment.

Artificial intelligence can be useful during an MRI examination, for example. MRI images consist of hundreds of thousands of individual image data in which neural networks recognize patterns and calculate the (6) _____ for certain diseases. To do this, they were previously trained with numerous MRI images and the associated diagnoses.

The AI supported assistance systems provide the doctor with important information for her own (7) _____. However, special skills are required to be able to deal with it in a reflective manner.

In summary, these two aspects are particularly important. On the one hand, AI systems must be trained with as much data as possible in order to deliver (8) _____ results. On the other hand, doctors need (9) _____ skills to be able to make better decisions in the interest of the patient supported by AI. In this way, the potential of artificial intelligence for medicine can be used in a reflective and (10) _____ manner.

VI. Pros/Cons Challenges for Big Data Application in Healthcare of China

1. **Read the following passage with ten statements attached to it. Each statement contains information given in one of the paragraphs. Identify the paragraph from which the information is derived. You may choose a paragraph more than once. Each paragraph is marked with a letter.**

_____ (1) Individual electronic health records with various technical structures and data standards are not effectively applied by different hospitals or healthcare systems.

_____ (2) "Medical migration" is also a problem in China due to the deficiency of an established referral system and the heterogeneity in the quality of healthcare.

_____ (3) Another problem with using big data in medical research is the inconsistency of medical terminology systems, which requires a general standard in the coding of clinical terms.

_____ (4) Problems can be solved if we examine the characteristics of the database and judge which variables are likely to be relatively accurate.

_____ (5) With its promotion of big data application in health and medicine, China manage to figure out the best way in the the development of the healthcare industry with traditional moral values.

_____ (6) Currently, a patient is not available to achieve his electronic record systems for clinical purposes because there is no specific national platform that can consolidate all the data from all healthcare institutions in China.

_____ (7) Electronic medical records in China are mostly applied in clinical practice and their data follows no strict standard.

_____ (8) Privacy should be supersized under specific law or guidance and privacy protection should not run in the opposite direction of the completeness of data.

_____ (9) The establishment of regional electronic health records should overcome a series of problems with the recognition from experts and professional institutions.

_____ (10) More effective and interoperable biomedical information systems and services should be applied to get full use of electronic health records in China.

Electronic Record Systems

A) Electronic medical records, whether collected by one organization or for individual patients across organizations, are not commonly used for research in China. They are primarily used for clinical practice and largely contain unstructured data. Although over 90% of hospitals in China use electronic records, accessibility to and quality of the data are not optimal.

B) Adoption of individual electronic health records has been impeded by incompatibility between different hospital systems. China has over 300 commercial providers of hospital information systems with various technical structures and data standards. Furthermore, healthcare systems are not required to exchange data with each other.

C) Some regions are planning to establish regional electronic health records but most are in preliminary stages. To overcome these problems, the interoperability of electronic records needs to be improved, especially for data structures, data standards, and data transfer agreements. Health authorities, hospitals, and electronic record companies must agree on how to improve hospital information systems. Technologies that can integrate data from different sources are also needed. In addition，the government should introduce policies to strengthen data exchange and integration across organizations.

Lack of Medical Terminology System

D）The lack of a widely adopted and consistently implemented medical terminology system is another problem with using big data in medical research. For example，since 2002，the use of the International Classification of Diseases（ICD‑9，and more recently ICD‑10）was mandated by the National Health and Family Planning Commission（now the National Health Commission）for all hospital patients. However，the growth of hospital information systems has resulted in many variations in the coding of other clinical terms beyond diagnosis，making data exchange difficult.

E）Widely accepted terminology systems，such as the Systematized Nomenclature of Medicine-Clinical Terms（SNOMED CT），the Unified Medical Language System（UMLS），or the General Architecture for Languages，Encyclopedias and Nomenclatures in Medicine（GALEN），are not available in China. By integrating and distributing key terminology，classification，and coding standards in medicine，these systems promote more effective and interoperable biomedical information systems and services，including electronic health records. More effort is needed to resolve linguistic differences between Chinese and English beyond the existing translation of terms.

Current Medical Practice Patterns

F）Medical practice patterns and the infrastructure of health systems in China also impede the meaningful use of big data. The lack of an established referral system and the heterogeneity in the quality of healthcare contribute to "medical migration"，when patients travel to different provinces and cities to seek medical care.

G）In the current Chinese medical system，it is almost impossible to track a patient through electronic record systems for clinical purposes as there is no unified national platform that can consolidate all the data from all healthcare institutions in China. The main barrier to conducting a "deep patient" study，where machine learning is used to predict future adverse events using medical data，is obtaining the longitudinal data and outcomes of each patient from electronic records. Furthermore，the wide differences in medical practice raise concerns about the veracity of data.

Data Quality

H）The problems described above affect the quality of big data. It has been shown that，when the quality of clinical data is higher，big data analytics produce more valid，stable，and clinically useful results. However，it is difficult to validate high volume data sets. One way of dealing with the data quality problem is to examine the characteristics of the database and judge which variables are likely to be relatively accurate — for example，expenditure from claims data — and to answer questions based on those variables. Improving the veracity of data requires an ongoing and joint effort by multiple sectors to rigorously examine the validity，representativeness，and completeness of data.

Privacy Concerns

I) Although privacy is an extremely important topic for big data in health and medicine, there is no specific law or guidance on this in China. Regulation from authorities and research standards about privacy protection are needed that do not jeopardize the completeness of data that can be used.

Conclusion

J) China's national campaign to promote the application of big data in health and medicine is likely to change medical research, medical practice, and the development of the healthcare industry in the near future. Despite the great interest in big data, we advocate following Confucian doctrine to ensure that we obtain true value for medicine — that is, to learn extensively, inquire carefully, think deeply, discriminate clearly, and practise faithfully.

2. Read the following statements. Decide to what extent you agree or disagree with each statement, and write your own pros or cons in the box, then set out your rational viewpoint and the reasons.

(1) The application of big data to health and medicine should be a national priority for China.

(2) Government should be more responsible for establishing initiatives to promote big data.

(3) The use of big data and new data technologies has the potential to improve medical research, and the understanding of health and disease.

(4) Individuals should also take the responsibility in the collection of big data in medicine.

(5) Application of big data should be available to all kinds of diseases.

Pros	Cons

VII. Outcome　Sentence Analysis and Essay Writing

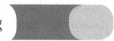

1. **Sentence-structure Analysis**

   Analyze the following sentences and draw a tree-structure.

   （1）Although difficult, it may be defined as a "cultural, technological, and scholarly phenomenon" based on the application of machine learning algorithms to data process and analysis.

   （2）We posit that this new perspective is endowed with unique opportunities, but also with menacing threats, which need to be promptly addressed, provided also the unparalleled intrusive capacity of new technologies.

   （3）The policy blueprint, which defined the country's spending priorities until 2020, pledged to "spur innovation and industrial application" in precision medicine alongside other areas such as smart vehicles and new materials.

2. **Essay Writing**

   Write an essay based on the picture. Search for relevant information and write at least 200 words. The following outline is for your reference.

   Outline：

   （1）What do you know about big data in medicine?

   （2）Introduce the devices and their functions to professional institutions and individuals.

   （3）Indicate the prospect of big data medicine in China.

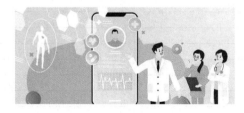

Unit 1

Unit 2

Unit 3

Unit 4

Unit 5

Unit 6

Unit 7

Unit 8

Unit 6
Pandemic

Web News on Pandemics

Read the web page. Then answer the questions orally.

Pandemics

| Prepare for Pandemic | Stay Safe During | Stay Safe After | Associated Content |

A pandemic is a disease outbreak that spans several countries and affects a large number of people. Pandemics are most often caused by viruses, which can easily spread from person to person.

A new virus can emerge from anywhere and quickly spread around the world. It is hard to predict when or where the next new pandemic will emerge.

If a Pandemic Is Declared

- Wash your hands often with soap and water for at least 20 seconds and try not to touch your eyes, nose or mouth.
- Keep a distance of at least six feet between yourself and people who are not part of your household.
- Cover your mouth and nose with a mask when in public.
- Clean and disinfect high-touch objects and surfaces.
- Stay at home as much as possible to prevent the spread of disease.
- Follow the guidance of the Centers for Disease Control and Prevention (CDC).

How to Prepare Yourself for a Pandemic

- Learn how diseases spread to help protect yourself and others. Viruses can be spread from person to person, from a nonliving object to a person and by people who are infected but don't have any symptoms.
- Prepare for the possibility of schools, workplaces and community centers being closed. Investigate and prepare for virtual coordination for school, work (telework) and social activities.

- Gather supplies in case you need to stay home for several days or weeks. Supplies may include cleaning supplies, nonperishable foods, prescriptions and bottled water. Buy supplies slowly to ensure that everyone has the opportunity to buy what they need.
- Create an emergency plan so that you and your family know what to do and what you will need in case an outbreak happens. Consider how a pandemic may affect your plans for other emergencies.
- Review your health insurance policies to understand what they cover, including telemedicine options.
- Create password-protected digital copies of important documents and store in a safe place. Watch out for scams and fraud.

Stay Safe During a Pandemic

- Take actions to prevent the spread of disease. Cover coughs and sneezes. Wear a mask in public. Stay home when sick (except to get medical care). Disinfect surfaces. Wash hands with soap and water for at least 20 seconds. If soap and water are not available, use a hand sanitizer that contains at least 60 percent alcohol.
- If you believe you've been exposed to the disease, contact your doctor, follow the quarantine instructions from medical providers and monitor your symptoms. If you're experiencing a medical emergency, call the emergency center and shelter in place with a mask, if possible, until help arrives.
- Share accurate information about the disease with friends, family and people on social media. Sharing bad information about the disease or treatments for the disease may have serious health outcomes. Remember that stigma hurts everyone and can cause discrimination against people, places or nations.
- Know that it's normal to feel anxious or stressed. Engage virtually with your community through video and phone calls. Take care of your body and talk to someone if you are feeling upset.

telemedicine [ˈtelɪˌmedɪsɪn]	*n.* the treatment of people who are ill, by sending information from one place to another by computer, video, etc. 远程医疗
scam [skæm]	*n.* a clever and dishonest plan for making money 欺诈; 诈骗
fraud [frɔːd]	*n.* a person who pretends to have qualities, abilities, etc. that they do not really have in order to cheat other people 骗子; 行骗的人
sanitizer [ˈsænɪtaɪzə(r)]	*n.* a liquid for washing your hands in order to get rid of harmful bacteria from them 食品防腐剂; 消毒杀菌剂

（1）As a student，what would you do to prepare yourself for a pandemic?

_____

（2）During a pandemic，how do you keep yourself safe?

_____

（3）What lessons will you learn from a pandemic?

_____

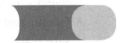

II. Watching-in Getting to know Pandemic

1. **View the video clips again. Match the photos（A－D）to the dialogues（1－4）. Then answer the following questions.**

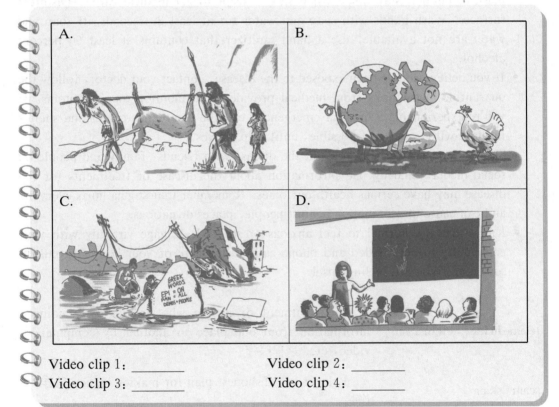

Video clip 1：_____   Video clip 2：_____
Video clip 3：_____   Video clip 4：_____

（1）How has globalization affected the spread of infectious diseases?

_____

（2）How do epidemics and pandemics occur，and what is an example of historical pandemic evidence?

_____

（3）What is the greatest pandemic killer and how does it typically mutate?

_____

2. **View the video clips again. Fill in the blanks to complete the sentences which can help you get the gist of the content.**

(1)

We live in an interconnected, an increasingly 1) _____ world. Thanks to international 2) _____, people and the diseases they carry can be in any city on the planet in a matter of hours. And once a virus 3) _____, sometimes all it takes is one 4) _____ to spread the infection throughout the community. When humans were hunter-gatherers, roaming the wild savannas, we were never in one place long enough, and settlements were not large enough to sustain the 5) _____ of infectious microbes. But with the advent of the 6) _____ 10,000 years ago, and the arrival of 7) _____ settlements in the Middle East, people began living side-by-side with animals, 8) _____ the spread of bacteria and viruses between cattle and humans.

(2)

Epidemics and pandemics come in many 1) _____. In 2010, for instance, a devastating earthquake struck Haiti, forcing thousands of people into 2) _____ refugee camps. Within weeks, the camps had become 3) _____ grounds for cholera, a bacteria spread by 4) _____ water, triggering a country-wide epidemic. But the most common cause of epidemics are viruses, such as measles, influenza and HIV. And when they go 5) _____, we call them pandemics. Pandemics have occurred throughout human history. Some have left scars on the tissue and bone of their 6) _____, while evidence for others comes from 7) _____ DNA. For instance, scientists have recovered DNA from the bacteria that transmits tuberculosis from the 8) _____ of ancient Egyptian mummies.

(3)

By far the greatest pandemic killer is influenza. Flu is constantly 1) _____ between the Southern and Northern Hemispheres. In North America and Europe, 2) _____ flus occur every autumn and winter. As the majority of children and adults will have been 3) _____ to the virus in previous seasons, these illnesses are usually 4) _____.

(4)

In terms of 1) _____, none can compare with the Great Flu Pandemic of 1918. An estimated 675,000 Americans and 230,000 Britons were dead. In India alone, some 10 million were killed, and worldwide the 2) _____ was an astonishing 50 million. But that was then. Today, planes can 3) _____ viruses to any country on the globe in

Unit 1 Unit 2 Unit 3 Unit 4 Unit 5 Unit 6 Unit 7 Unit 8

However，every 20 to 40 years or so the virus undergoes a dramatic 5) _____ . Usually this occurs when a wild flu virus circulating in ducks and farm poultry meets a pig virus，and they 6) _____ genes. This process is known as 7) _____ and has occurred throughout human history. The first 8) _____ pandemic occurred in 1580. The 18th and 19th centuries saw at least six further pandemics.

a 4) _____ of the time it took in 1918. If history teaches us anything, it's that while pandemics may start 5) _____ , their impacts can be as 6) _____ as wars and natural disasters. The difference today is that science gives us the ability to 7) _____ pandemics right at the very beginning and to take action to 8) _____ their impacts before they spread too widely.

jet [dʒet]	*n*. a plane driven by jet engines 喷气式飞机
sneeze [sniːz]	*v*. to have air come suddenly and noisily out through your nose and mouth in a way that you cannot control，for example because you have a cold 打喷嚏
savanna [sə'vænə]	*n*. a large，flat area of land covered with grass, usually with few trees，that is found in hot countries, especially in Africa 热带大草原
antigenic ['æntɪdʒenɪk]	*adj*. relating to or consisting of antigens（＝ substances that cause the body's immune system to react，especially causing it to produce antibodies）抗原的
toll [təʊl]	*n*. the amount of damage or the number of deaths and injuries that are caused in a particular war, disaster，etc.（战争、灾难等造成的）毁坏；伤亡人数
mitigate ['mɪtɪɡeɪt]	*v*. to make sth less harmful，serious，etc. 减轻；缓和

III. Leading-in Defining Pandemic

1. **View a video clip and fill in the blanks. Then define the term "pandemic" in your own words.**

What is a pandemic? A pandemic is the (1) _____ spread of a new disease. The Flu of 1918 is considered to be one of the (2) _____ pandemics in human history. It (3) _____ more than 500 million people. Pandemics are (4) _____ classified as epidemics first. An epidemic is a disease that (5) _____ many people within a community, population or region. An epidemic becomes a pandemic when it spreads to (6) _____ countries or continents. The Zika virus outbreak as well as the Ebola outbreak are both (7) _____ as epidemics. An influenza pandemic occurs when a new influenza virus against which people do not have (8) _____ emerges and spreads around the world. In the past, pandemics have been caused by viruses which have typically (9) _____ from animal influenza viruses.

2. **Read the following passage and answer these questions.**

(1) Why aren't cancer and seasonal influenza considered pandemics?

_____

_____

(2) According to the research, what are the reasons for the four historic influenza pandemics?

_____

_____

(3) Why was smallpox eradicated worldwide in 1979?

_____

_____

Passage A

Overview of Pandemic

A pandemic is an epidemic of an infectious disease that has spread across a large region, for instance, multiple continents or worldwide, affecting a substantial number of people. A disease or condition is not a pandemic merely because it is widespread or kills many people; it must also be infectious. For instance, cancer is respon-

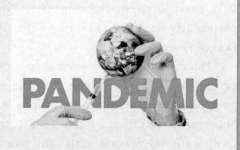

sible for many deaths but is not considered a pandemic because the disease is not contagious (i. e. easily transmittable) and not even simply infectious. A widespread endemic disease with a stable number of infected people is not a pandemic. Widespread endemic diseases with a stable number of infected people such as recurrences of seasonal influenza are generally excluded as they occur simultaneously in large regions of the globe rather than being spread worldwide.

Throughout human history, there have been a number of pandemics of diseases as follows:

HIV/AIDS

HIV originated in Africa and spread to the United States via Haiti between 1966 and 1972. AIDS is currently a pandemic in Africa, with infection rates as high as 25% in some regions of southern and eastern Africa. In 2006, the HIV prevalence among pregnant women in South Africa was 29%. Effective education about safer sexual practices and bloodborne infection precautions training has helped to slow down infection rates in several African countries sponsoring national education programs. There were an estimated 1.5 million new infections of HIV/AIDS in 2020. As of 2020, there have been about a total of 32.7 million deaths related to HIV/AIDS since the epidemic started.

Black Death

The total number of deaths worldwide is estimated at 75 million to 200 million. Eight hundred years after the last outbreak, the plague returned to Europe. In six years since 1348, the disease killed an estimated 20 million to 30 million Europeans, a third of the total population, and up to a half in the worst-affected urban areas. It was the first of a cycle of European plague epidemics that continued until the 18th century. The disease recurred in England every two to five years from 1361 to 1480. By the 1370s, England's population was reduced by 50%. The Great Plague of London of 1665 – 1666 was the last major outbreak of the plague in England and killed approximately 100,000 people, 20% of London's population.

Cholera

A disease of the large intestine and transmitted through contaminated water, cholera has haunted humanity for centuries. This cholera pandemic is considered the most deadly cholera pandemic in history. The third cholera pandemic from 1852 to 1859 swept through Asia, North America, and Africa, hitting Russia particularly hard and caused 1 million Russian deaths.

Dengue Fever

Dengue is spread by several species of female mosquitoes of the Aedes type, principally A. aegypti. The virus has five types; infection with one type usually gives lifelong immunity to that type, but only short-term immunity to the others. Subsequent infection with a different type increases the risk of severe complications. Several tests are available to confirm the diagnosis including detecting antibodies to the virus or its RNA.

Influenza

The first influenza pandemic to be pathologically described occurred in 1510. Since the pandemic of 1580, influenza pandemics have occurred every 10 to 30 years. The influenza pandemic of 1918 – 1919, so-called the Flu of 1918, was the most destructive influenza outbreak in history, during which an estimated 25 million persons throughout the world died. The latest outbreak of swine flu occurred in 2009, which first broke out in Mexico and then spread to the United States. Research has indicated that each of the four historic influenza pandemics was preceded by a La Niña event — a change in global weather conditions associated with cool sea surface temperatures in the Pacific Ocean — which, some scientists speculate, may have altered the migratory patterns of birds, possibly increasing their interactions with domestic animals and enabling genetic reassortment and the rise of new pandemic strains of influenza viruses.

Smallpox

Smallpox was a contagious disease caused by the variola virus. The disease killed an estimated 400,000 Europeans per year during the closing years of the 18th century. During the 20th century, it is estimated that smallpox was responsible for 300 million – 500 million deaths. As recently as the early 1950s, an estimated 50 million cases of smallpox occurred in the world each year. After successful vaccination campaigns throughout the 19th and 20th centuries, the WHO certified the eradication of smallpox in December 1979. To this day, smallpox is the only human infectious disease to have been completely eradicated, and one of two infectious viruses ever to be eradicated, along with rinderpest.

Tuberculosis

One-quarter of the world's current population has been infected with Mycobacterium tuberculosis, and new infections occur at a rate of one per second. About 5%- 10% of these latent infections will eventually progress to active disease, which, if left untreated, kills more than half its victims. Annually, eight million people become ill with tuberculosis, and two million die from the disease worldwide. In the 19th century, tuberculosis killed an estimated one-quarter of the adult population of Europe; by 1918, one in six deaths in France were still caused by tuberculosis. During the 20th century, tuberculosis killed approximately 100 million people. TB is still one of the most important health problems in the developing world. In 2018, tuberculosis becomes the leading cause of death from an infectious disease, with roughly 1.5 million deaths worldwide.

Malaria

Malaria is widespread in tropical and subtropical regions, including parts of the Americas, Asia, and Africa. Each year, there are approximately 350 million – 500 million cases of malaria. Drug resistance poses a growing problem in the treatment of malaria in the 21st century, since resistance is now common against all classes of antimalarial drugs, except for the artemisinins. During the American

Civil War, there were more than 1.2 million cases of malaria among soldiers of both sides. The southern US continued to be afflicted with millions of cases of malaria into the 1930s.

endemic [en'demɪk]	*adj*. (esp. of diseases) found regularly in a particular place (指疾病)地方性的
recurrence [rɪ'kʌrəns]	*n*. the fact of happening again 复发
precaution [prɪ'kɔːʃən]	*n*. an action taken in advance to protect against possible danger, failure, or injury 预防措施
contaminate [kən'tæmɪneɪt]	*v*. to make impure or unsuitable by contact or mixture with sth unclean, bad, etc.; pollute 感染,污染
dengue fever ['deŋgɪ'fiːvə(r)]	*n*. an infectious disease of the tropics transmitted by mosquitoes and characterized by rash and aching head and joints 登革热
complication [ˌkɒmplɪ'keɪʃən]	*n*. a new problem or illness that makes treatment of a previous one more complicated or difficult 并发症
pathologically [ˌpæθə'lɒdʒɪkəlɪ]	*adv*. with respect to pathology 病理上;与疾病相关
swine [swaɪn]	*n*. (old use or tech) a pig (旧用法或技术)猪
reassortment [ˌriːə'sɔːtmənt]	*n*. (genetics) the formation of a hybrid virus containing parts from the genomes of two distinct viruses in a mixed infection (病毒基因)重组
variola [və'raɪələ]	*n*. smallpox 天花;痘疮

3. **Match each of the terms listed below with the numbered definition. Write the letter in the space provided.**

A. tuberculosis	E. acute	I. epidemic
B. immunity	F. complication	J. outbreak
C. contamination	G. infection	K. contagious
D. respiratory	H. fatality	L. vaccine

(1) _____ : any disease or disorder that occurs during the course of (or because of) another disease

(2) _____ : (of a disease) that can be spread by touch or through the air

(3) _____ : the sudden start of sth unpleasant, especially violence or a disease

(4) _____ : immunogen consisting of a suspension of weakened or dead pathogenic cells injected in order to stimulate the production of antibodies

(5) _____ : (of a disease) the invasion of the body by pathogenic microorganisms and their multiplication which can lead to tissue damage and disease

(6) _____ : a communicable disease caused by infection with the tubercle bacillus, most frequently affecting the lungs

(7) _____ : connected with breathing

(8) _____ : the presence of an unwanted constituent, contaminant or impurity in a material, physical body, natural environment, workplace, etc

(9) _____ : deadly effect; deadliness

(10) _____ : resistance to or protection against a specified disease

(11) _____ : (of a disease) coming quickly to a dangerous condition

(12) _____ : a widespread occurrence of a disease

IV. Critical Reading Further Reading on Pandemics

1. **Influenza Transmission and Precaution**

Read the following passage and complete the exercises that follow.

A. Fill in the blanks to complete the table.

Item	Factor
Transmission of influenza	A respiratory virus carried by (1) _____ infects people through (2) _____ into lungs and exposure through (3) _____ . Prevalence of influenza occurs during (4) _____ .
Precautions of the spread	Avoiding (5) _____ . (6) _____ can slow down influenza infection rates. Besides (7) _____ , taking (8) _____ drugs and having good (9) _____ can help prevent the spread of the flu and other respiratory illnesses.

B. Judge whether the statements are true (T) or false (F).

_____ (1) Hand washing is unable to reduce the spread of the virus during the height of their infection.

_____ (2) Children spread influenza more efficiently than do adults.

_____ (3) It's safe to share cups and utensils with infected individuals, and it will not increases the risk of infection.

_____ (4) Among the three types of influenza, Influenza B produces more serious cases of illness.

_____ (5) Vaccination prevents the spread of influenza in common forms, but it does not guarantee protection from the spread of new mutations.

Passage B
Influenza Transmission and Precaution

Influenza is an infectious respiratory virus spread by aerosol droplets emitted by those infected. Infection comes from direct inhalation into the lungs and exposure through the nose and mouth. The spread of influenza from one person to another can occur even before infected individuals experience flu symptoms, but is worst during the height of fever. Children spread influenza more efficiently than do adults. The virus needs moisture and will dry out quickly if exposed to ultraviolet radiation or dry air, which may account for the prevalence of influenza during humid and darker winter weather.

In moist droplets, the influenza virus can survive outside of the body for a time on things like railings, dishes, and doorknobs. Through these it is spread by hand-to-mouth contact when someone touches an object contaminated with the aerosols and then touches his or her own mouth. Sharing cups and utensils with infected individuals increases the risk of infection. For this reason, consistent hand washing with soap and water and properly washing dishes and utensils helps reduce the spread of influenza.

Two major factors in the spread of influenza depend on the strain of the virus and its rate of mutation, since flu strains constantly mutate as they compete with host immune systems. Influenza B and C are milder forms, but influenza A produces more serious cases of illness. Pandemics occur when a virulent strain of flu infects millions of people around the world, typically due to new mutations that have migrated from other animals to humans. The 1918 Flu outbreak, for instance, resulted from a mutated strain related to avian influenza that caused hemorrhage and other unusually severe symptoms.

The three kinds of influenza spread at different rates, but the all of them are spread through the coughing and sneezing of infected individuals. Hygienic precautions like hand washing and avoiding proximity to sick people during the height of their infection reduces the spread of the virus. Vaccination can slow down influenza infection rates and protect vulnerable populations.

Vaccination prevents the spread of influenza in common forms, particularly of influenza B, but it does not guarantee protection from the spread of new mutations. It is recommended for the elderly, who are at greater risk of serious complications.

While how well the flu vaccine works can vary, there are a lot of reasons to get a flu vaccine each year.

- Flu vaccination can keep you from getting sick with flu.
- Flu vaccination can reduce the risk of flu-associated hospitalization, including among children and older adults.

  a. A 2014 study showed that flu vaccine reduced children's risk of flu-related pediatric intensive care unit (PICU) admission by 74% during flu seasons from 2010 – 2012.

  b. Another study published in the summer of 2016 showed that people 50 years and older who got a flu vaccine reduced their risk of getting hospitalized from the flu by 57%.

- Flu vaccination is an important preventive tool for people with chronic health conditions.

  a. Vaccination was associated with lower rates of some cardiac events among people with heart disease, especially among those who had had a cardiac event in the past year.

  b. Flu vaccination also has been shown to be associated with reduced hospitalization among people with diabetes (79%) and chronic lung disease (52%).

- Vaccination helps protect women during and after pregnancy. Getting vaccinated can also protect a baby after birth from flu. (Mom passes antibodies onto the developing baby during her pregnancy.)

  a. A study that looked at flu vaccine effectiveness in pregnant women found that vaccination reduced the risk of flu-associated acute respiratory infection by about one half.

  b. There are studies that show that flu vaccine in a pregnant woman can reduce the risk of flu illness in her baby by up to half. This protective benefit was observed for up to four months after birth.

- Flu vaccination also may make your illness milder if you do get sick.

Getting vaccinated yourself also protects people around you, including those who are more vulnerable to serious flu illness, like babies and young children, older people, and people with certain chronic health conditions. If flu sufferers rest at home and avoid public places until recovery, they are less likely to expose others to the virus.

Getting a flu vaccine each year is the best way to prevent the flu. Antiviral drugs are an important second line of defense against the flu. These drugs must be prescribed by a doctor. In addition, good health habits, such as covering your cough and frequently washing your hands with soap, can help prevent the spread of the flu and other respiratory illnesses.

aerosol [ˈeərəʊsɒl]	*n.* a cloud of solid or liquid particles in a gas 气溶胶
droplet [ˈdrɒplɪt]	*n.* a tiny drop 小水滴
inhalation [ˌɪnhəˈleɪʃən]	*n.* the act of inhaling; breathing in air or other vapours 吸入
ultraviolet [ˌʌltrəˈvaɪələt]	*adj.* lying outside the visible spectrum at its violet end 紫外线的
humid [ˈhjuːmɪd]	*adj.* containing or characterized by a high amount of water or water vapor 潮湿的
utensil [juːˈtensəl]	*n.* a tool that is used in the house 器皿，家什
mutated [mjuːˈteɪtɪd]	*adj.* physically different from other plants or animals of the same type as a result of a genetic change 变异的；突变的
avian [ˈeɪvɪən]	*adj.* of or connected with birds 鸟类的
hemorrhage [ˈhemərɪdʒ]	*n.* excessive discharge of blood; profuse bleeding 大出血
hygienic [haɪˈdʒiːnɪk]	*adj.* clean and free of bacteria and therefore unlikely to spread disease 卫生的
proximity [prɒkˈsɪmətɪ]	*n.* nearness or closeness in space or time 接近
hospitalization [ˌhɒspɪtəlaɪˈzeɪʃən]	*n.* the act of placing a person in a hospital as a patient 住院

2. Controversial Bird-Flu Research Published：How Worried Should We Be？

Read the following passage to fill in the blanks，and then check your understanding.

A controversial research paper was released：

The paper shows that（1）_____ has the potential to become a human pandemic. The research demonstrates an experiment on （2）_____ with the H1N1 pandemic virus of 2009. The research reveals the current H5N1 virus would become（3）_____ and it could turn into a worrisome human pathogen.

Controversy aroused on the research of bird flu virus' transmissibility：

a. Disagreement on this research，many biosecurity experts believe（4）_____ _____，and that the world would be a safer place if information about the results of the Kawaoka and Fouchier experiments and their methods were never disseminated.

b. Standing strongly，many scientists believe（5）_____ _____ is too urgent to be put under onerous security constraints，even

though the research that (6) _____ certainly
pose a risk.

Question left: Which should we fear most?

Risk of (7) _____ or danger of (8) ____

_____?

Passage C

Controversial Bird-Flu Research Published: How Worried Should We Be?

A highly controversial research paper on bird flu was released today by the journal *Nature*. It shows that a particularly troublesome strain of avian influenza, designated H5N1, which has been worrying public health officials for more than a decade, has the potential to become a human pandemic. In other words, H5N1 bird flu, which so far has been highly lethal to humans but has not acquired the ability to spread easily among us, could do so at any time.

The researchers, under the direction of Yoshihiro Kawaoka at the University of Wisconsin at Madison, crossed an H5N1 virus with the H1N1 pandemic virus of 2009, which spread like wildfire from one end of the world to another. The 2009 pandemic, you'll recall, caught public health officials by surprise but luckily turned out to be mild. Kawaoka's lab-made hybrid virus spreads among ferrets by airborne droplets expelled during the course of respiration — just as human influenza viruses such as the 2009 pandemic strain spread from person to person. Kawaoka's concoction does not kill ferrets, and probably wouldn't kill humans, but the feat is troubling because it demonstrates that an H5N1 virus that can spread among humans is most likely possible. (We don't know for sure because it was tested only on ferrets, not humans, of course.)

The known H5N1 viruses that currently exist in nature do not attach to the upper respiratory tracts of humans, so most victims caught the virus from close contact with birds. And there is reason to think that a highly lethal but poorly transmissible virus like H5N1 would change in the process of becoming transmissible — that in acquiring the ability to spread, the virus would have to make genetic tradeoffs that compromise its ability to kill. For instance, one reason that the Ebola virus doesn't spread widely among humans is that it is too efficient — mortality is as high as 90 percent — which means victims die before they can infect many others. We do not know, however, to what extent a human-transmissible H5N1 virus would have to make this tradeoff. Scientists differ widely in their opinions on this point.

The strain that Kawaoka concocted in his lab seems to be mild — it made ferrets sick, but didn't kill them. Even if this virus is not itself dangerous, however, it demonstrates that an H5N1 strain could one day arise that turns into a worrisome human pathogen. As Michael Osterholm, director of the Center for Infectious Disease Research and Policy at the University of Minnesota, has pointed out, a human-transmissible virus with a lethality rate 20 times lower than current wild strains of H5N1 would still kill more efficiently than the 1918 flu. The degree to which H5N1 is potentially dangerous to humans is the subject of much speculation.

In part because of all the uncertainty, the biosecurity community has been in an uproar ever since the Kawaoka paper came to their attention last year. (Things really got stirred up when Ron Fouchier of Erasmus Medical Center in Rotterdam made remarks at a conference in Malta about similar work on H5N1 transmissibility, which he submitted to *Science* but has been held up by the Dutch government.) Many security experts believe no work on H5N1 transmissibility among mammals should have been conducted in the first place, and that the world would be a safer place if information about the results of the Kawaoka and Fouchier experiments and their methods were never disseminated. (Although the National Science Advisory Board for Biosecurity voted to green-light the publication of both papers, that vote came only after the results and the methods used to make the viruses had been disseminated to hundreds of people in the course of the standard prepublication review process; holding up publication at that point, in this age of Wikileaks, probably would have been futile.) Recently the US government has called for risk-benefit assessments of pathogens on its select agent list before research is conducted (H5N1 is on that list), but compliance is left to the funding agencies. Some biosecurity experts are calling for further restrictions in H5N1 research on transmissibility among mammals, such as limiting the work to labs with the highest biosafety standards.

Many scientists believe this would be a mistake. They think that research on what could possibly make H5N1 deadly to humans is too urgent to be put under onerous security constraints. Kawaoka was interviewed in 2010, during the course of research for the book, *The Fate of the Species* (which Bloomsbury releases on May 22). At the time, Kawaoka was deeply worried about the danger of H5N1 bird flu. There had been outbreaks among poultry in 1997 and again in 2004 in Asia, and the virus had shown other signs of restlessness — it had killed wild birds, which usually carry H5N1 without symptoms, and it had shown a propensity to spread outward from east Asia, despite the culling of millions of chickens and other poultry. How long would it be before nature's roulette wheel produced a human version of H5N1?

Researchers so far have already found natural strains of H5N1 that have acquired some of the genetic changes that Kawaoka's recent paper identifies as necessary for transmissibility among ferrets. The research that Kawaoka and other influenza scientists are conducting certainly poses a risk, as some biosecurity experts have pointed out. The experiment reveals that nature is conducting every day, as H5N1 viruses mutate and borrow genetic material from other viruses, which is also potentially dangerous. Which should we fear most? On this question there are many opinions, but no definitive answers.

controversial [ˌkɒntrəˈvɜːʃəl]	*adj*. causing a lot of angry public discussion and disagreement 有争议的
designate [ˈdezɪgneɪt]	*v*. to say officially that sb/sth has a particular character or name 命名，指定
lethal [ˈliːθəl]	*adj*. causing or able to cause death 致命的
hybrid [ˈhaɪbrɪd]	*adj*. bred from two distinct races, breeds, varieties, or species 杂交的
ferret [ˈferɪt]	*n*. a small aggressive animal with a long thin body, kept for chasing rabbits from their holes, killing rats, etc 白鼬
respiration [ˌrespəˈreɪʃən]	*n*. the act of breathing 呼吸
tradeoff [ˈtreɪdɒf]	*n*. an exchange of one thing in return for another 交易；权衡
concoct [kənˈkɒkt]	*v*. to make by combining different ingredients 调制
speculation [ˌspekjʊˈleɪʃn]	*n*. the act of forming opinions about what has happened or what might happen without knowing all the facts 推测，猜测
disseminate [dɪˈsemɪneɪt]	*v*. to scatter or spread widely 传播
futile [ˈfjuːtaɪl]	*adj*. incapable of producing any result；ineffective；useless；not successful 无效的，徒劳的
compliance [kəmˈplaɪəns]	*n*. the practice of obeying rules or requests made by people in authority 服从，顺从
onerous [ˈɒnərəs]	*adj*. needing great effort；causing trouble or worry 费力的；艰巨的
constraint [kənˈstreɪnt]	*n*. strict control over the way that you behave or are allowed to behave 约束，限制

3. **Lexical chunks and sentence rewriting.**

   A. Substitute the underlined part with the words or expressions you have learned.

   (1) Effective education about safer sexual practices and bloodborne infection precautions training have helped to <u>slow down</u> infection rates in several African countries sponsoring national education programs. (Passage A)

   Answer:

   Effective education about safer sexual practices and bloodborne infection precautions training have helped to _____ infection rates in several African countries sponsoring national education programs.

   (2) <u>As of</u> 2020 there have been about a total of 32.7 million deaths related to HIV/AIDS since the epidemic started. (Passage A)

   Answer:

   _____ 2020 there have been about a total of 32.7 million deaths related to HIV/AIDS since the epidemic started.

   (3) Drug resistance <u>poses a growing problem</u> in the treatment of malaria in the 21st century. (Passage A)

   Answer:

   Drug resistance _____ in malaria treatment in the 21st century.

   (4) The southern US continued to <u>be afflicted with</u> millions of cases of malaria into the 1930s. (Passage A)

   Answer:

   Until the 1930s, _____ still millions of malaria cases in the southern United States.

   (5) Influenza <u>spreads</u> around the world in a yearly outbreak, resulting in about three to five million cases of severe illness and about 250,000 to 500,000 deaths. (Passage B)

   Answer:

   Influenza _____ around the world in a yearly outbreak,……

   (6) …the 1918 influenza actually had a positive <u>long-term</u> effect on per-capita income growth,… (Passage B)

   Answer:

   …the 1918 influenza actually had a positive _____ effect on per-capita income growth,…

   (7) Sharing cups and utensils with infected individuals <u>increases</u> the risk of infection. (Passage B)

   Answer:

   Sharing cups and utensils with infected individuals _____ the risk of infection.

   (8) The 1918 Flu outbreak, for instance, <u>resulted from</u> a mutated strain related to avian influenza that caused hemorrhage and other unusually severe symptoms. (Passage B)

   Answer:

   The 1918 Flu outbreak, for instance, _____ a mutated strain related to avian influenza ......

(9) Vaccination was <u>associated</u> with lower rates of some cardiac events among people with heart disease, ... (Passage B)

Answer:

Vaccination was _____ with lower rates of some cardiac events among people with heart disease, ...

(10) A highly controversial research paper on bird flu was <u>released</u> today by the journal *Nature*. (Passage C)

Answer:

A highly controversial research paper on bird flu was _____ today by the journal *Nature*.

(11) The 2009 pandemic <u>caught</u> public health officials by surprise but luckily turned out to be mild. (Passage C)

Answer:

The 2009 pandemic _____ public health officials by surprise but luckily turned out to be mild.

(12) The feat is troubling because it <u>demonstrates</u> that an H5N1 virus that can spread among humans is most likely possible. (Passage C)

Answer:

The feat is troubling because it _____ that an H5N1 virus that can spread among humans is most likely possible.

(13) There is reason to think that a highly lethal but poorly transmissible virus like H5N1 would <u>change</u> in the process of becoming transmissible. (Passage C)

Answer:

There is reason to think that a highly lethal but poorly transmissible virus like H5N1 would _____ in the process of becoming transmissible.

B. Rewrite the following sentences using the academic expressions you have learned in the articles.

(1) Influenza is an infectious respiratory virus spread by aerosol droplets released from those infected.

Lexical chunks: _____

Sentence rewriting: _____

_____

(2) Vaccination correlated with lower rates of some cardiac events among people with heart disease, especially among those who had experienced a cardiac event in the past year.

Lexical chunks: _____

Sentence rewriting: _____

_____

(3) You may recall that the 2009 pandemic made public health officials surprised, but fortunately the results were mild.

Lexical chunks: _____

Sentence rewriting：_____

(4) Things really become complex when Ron Fouchier of Erasmus Medical Center in Rotterdam made remarks at a conference in Malta about similar work on H5N1 transmissibility.

Lexical chunks：_____

Sentence rewriting：_____

(5) ... and that the world would be a safer place if information about the results of the Kawaoka and Fouchier experiments and their methods were never spread.

Lexical chunks：_____

Sentence rewriting：_____

4. **Bilingual Translation**

Put the following into Chinese or vice versa.

A. English-Chinese translation

Learn the following useful expressions by translating the sentences from the passages.

(1) slow down (使)慢下来

Excerpt：

Vaccination can slow down influenza infection rates and protect vulnerable populations.

Translation：_____

(2) account for 说明(原因、理由等)；导致，引起

Excerpt：

The virus needs moisture and will dry out quickly if exposed to ultraviolet radiation or dry air，which may account for the prevalence of influenza during humid and darker winter weather.

Translation：_____

(3) guarantee ... from 保证……不……

Excerpt：

Vaccination prevents the spread of influenza in common forms，particularly of influenza B，but it does not guarantee protection from the spread of new mutations.

Translation：_____

(4) attach to (使)贴或粘在……上；(使)相关；(使)牵连

Excerpt：

The known H5N1 viruses that currently exist in nature do not attach to the upper respiratory tracts of humans, so most victims caught the virus from close contact with birds.

Translation：

_____

_____

（5）turn into（使）变成；成为

Excerpt：

Even if this virus is not itself dangerous, however, it demonstrates that an H5N1 strain could one day arise that turns into a worrisome human pathogen.

Translation：

_____

_____

（6）come to one's attention 成为……的关注点

Excerpt：

In part because of all the uncertainty, the biosecurity community has been in an uproar ever since the Kawaoka paper came to their attention last year.

Translation：

_____

_____

（7）call for 发起，号召

Excerpt：

Recently the US government has called for risk-benefit assessments of pathogens on its select agent list before research is conducted（H5N1 is on that list）, but compliance is left to the funding agencies.

Translation：

_____

_____

B. Chinese-English translation

Put the Chinese paragraph into English.

流感是通过空气飞沫或直接接触患者唾液、鼻腔分泌物而感染的呼吸道传染病。常见症状有发烧、头痛、全身酸痛、鼻塞、流涕、喉咙痛、咳嗽和疲倦无力。大部分患者可在一星期内痊愈，但是老年人及慢性病患者（如心脏病患者、慢性呼吸道疾病患者）则有可能出现并发症，甚至导致死亡。预防措施包括每年接种流感疫苗；日常饮食保持清淡且营养均衡，多吃新鲜水果、蔬菜；适量运动，保证充足睡眠。如出现流感症状，应戴上口罩避免传染他人并且及时就医；避免去人多拥挤的公共场合，在家休息，做好自我隔离。

_____

_____

_____

_____

Knowledge About Pandemic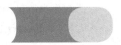

1. Read and say

Read the following comics. Work in pairs and fill in the blanks. Try to tell the story after you have completed the comic strips.

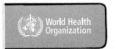

Monster Alert

A story of how we must act globally to protect ourselves locally from COVID-19

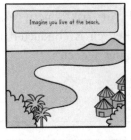

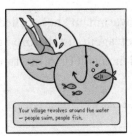

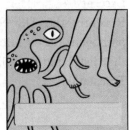

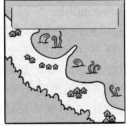

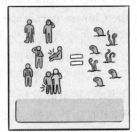

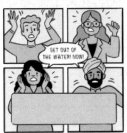

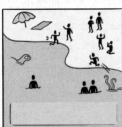

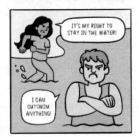

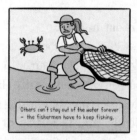

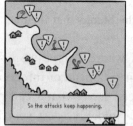

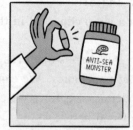

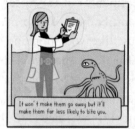

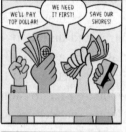

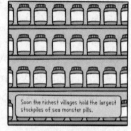

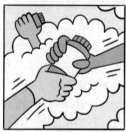

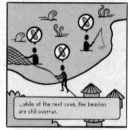

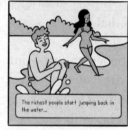

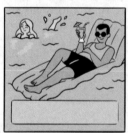

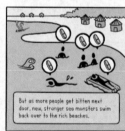

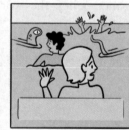

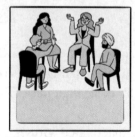

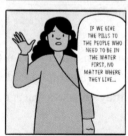

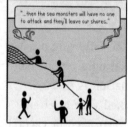

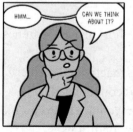

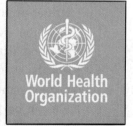

173

2. Watch and Act

Watch a video clip. Fill in the blanks and then act it out in class.

But there's one area where I hope we never go back: Our (1) _____ about pandemics. We can get ahead of infectious-disease outbreaks. By the next pandemic, I believe we can have what I call megatesting diagnostic platforms. They can be (2) _____ quickly, cost very little, and test 20% of the entire population every week. We also want to get treatments out far faster next time. One of the most (3) _____ is monoclonal antibodies. These manufactured antibodies grab onto the virus and disable it, just like your immune system and can reduce death rates by as much as 80%. I also think that we'll develop new (4) _____ quickly, in large part due to this new mRNA platform. mRNA will become faster to develop, easier to store, and lower cost. That's a huge (5) _____. To stop future pandemics quickly, we need to be able to (6) _____ disease outbreaks as soon as they happen anywhere in the world. And that requires a global (7) _____ system. If there turns out to be some new infectious (8) _____, then we need a group of infectious-disease responders to spring into action. Think of these as like pandemic (9) _____. They're going to use their logistics, use their ability to build up capacity quickly. They're going to go wherever that problem is. Stopping the next pandemic will require a big (10) _____. But I think of this as the best insurance policy the world could buy. You can read more about this in our annual letter.

VI. Pros/Cons Flu Vaccine

1. Read the following passage with ten statements attached to it. Each statement contains information given in one of the paragraphs. Identify the paragraph from which the information is derived. You may choose a paragraph more than once. Each paragraph is marked with a letter.

_____ (1) Flu vaccines are either made with inactivated viruses or with no flu viruses at all.

_____ (2) Common side effects of the flu shot include soreness, redness, or swelling at the injection site.

_____ (3) For the 2016 – 2017 flu season, the inactivated influenza vaccine or the recombinant influenza vaccine is recommended.

_____ (4) Flu can be particularly serious for young children, older adults, and people with certain chronic health conditions.

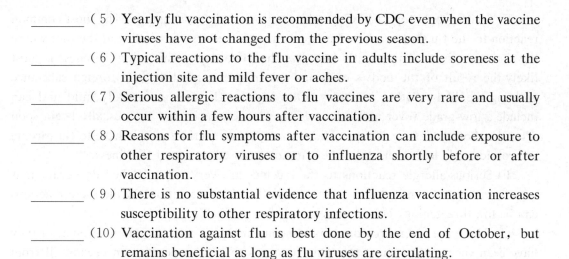

_____ (5) Yearly flu vaccination is recommended by CDC even when the vaccine viruses have not changed from the previous season.

_____ (6) Typical reactions to the flu vaccine in adults include soreness at the injection site and mild fever or aches.

_____ (7) Serious allergic reactions to flu vaccines are very rare and usually occur within a few hours after vaccination.

_____ (8) Reasons for flu symptoms after vaccination can include exposure to other respiratory viruses or to influenza shortly before or after vaccination.

_____ (9) There is no substantial evidence that influenza vaccination increases susceptibility to other respiratory infections.

_____ (10) Vaccination against flu is best done by the end of October, but remains beneficial as long as flu viruses are circulating.

A) A flu shot cannot cause flu illness. Flu vaccines given with a needle are currently made in two ways: The vaccine is made either with a) flu vaccine viruses that have been "inactivated" and are therefore not infectious, or b) with no flu vaccine viruses at all (which is the case for recombinant influenza vaccine). The most common side effects from the influenza shot are soreness, redness, tenderness or swelling where the shot was given. Low-grade fever, headache and muscle aches also may occur. In randomized, blinded studies, where some people get inactivated flu shots and others get salt-water shots, the only differences in symptoms was increased soreness in the arm and redness at the injection site among people who got the flu shot. There were no differences in terms of body aches, fever, cough, runny nose or sore throat.

B) For the 2016 – 2017 flu season, the Advisory Committee on Immunization Practices (ACIP) recommends annual influenza vaccination for everyone 6 months and older with either the inactivated influenza vaccine (IIV) or the recombinant influenza vaccine (RIV). The nasal spray flu vaccine (live attenuated influenza vaccine or LAIV) should not be used during 2016 – 2017. There is no preference for one vaccine over another among the recommended, approved injectable influenza vaccines. There are many vaccine options to choose from, but the most important thing is for all people 6 months and older to get a flu vaccine every year. If you have questions about which vaccine is best for you, talk to your doctor or other healthcare professional.

C) Flu can be a serious disease, particularly among young children, older adults, and people with certain chronic health conditions, such as asthma, heart disease or diabetes. Any flu infection can carry a risk of serious complications, hospitalization or death, even among otherwise healthy children and adults.

D) CDC recommends a yearly flu vaccine for just about everyone 6 months and older, even when the viruses the vaccine protects against have not changed from the previous season. The reason for this is that a person's immune protection from vaccination declines over time, so an annual vaccination is needed to get the "optimal" or best protection against the flu.

E) Some people report having mild reactions to flu vaccination. The most common reaction to the flu shot in adults has been soreness, redness or swelling at the spot where the shot was given. This usually lasts less than two days. This initial soreness is most likely the result of the body's early immune response reacting to a foreign substance entering the body. Other reactions following the flu shot are usually mild and can include a low-grade fever and aches. If these reactions occur, they usually begin soon after the shot and last 1 - 2 days. The most common reactions people have to flu vaccine are considerably less severe than the symptoms caused by actual flu illness.

F) Serious allergic reactions to flu vaccines are very rare. If they do occur, it is usually within a few minutes to a few hours after the vaccination. While these reactions can be life-threatening, effective treatments are available.

G) There are several reasons why someone might get a flu symptom, even after they have been vaccinated against flu. One reason is that some people can become ill from other respiratory viruses besides flu such as rhinoviruses, which are associated with the common cold, cause symptoms similar to flu, and also spread and cause illness during the flu season. The flu vaccine only protects against influenza, not other illnesses. Another explanation is that it is possible to be exposed to influenza viruses, which cause the flu, shortly before getting vaccinated or during the two-week period after vaccination that it takes the body to develop immune protection. This exposure may result in a person becoming ill with flu before protection from the vaccine takes effect. A third reason why some people may experience flu-like symptoms despite getting vaccinated is that they may have been exposed to a flu virus that is very different from the viruses the vaccine is designed to protect against. The ability of a flu vaccine to protect a person depends largely on the similarity or "match" between the viruses selected to make the vaccine and those spreading and causing illness. There are many different flu viruses that spread and cause illness among people.

H) In adults, studies have not shown a benefit from getting more than one dose of vaccine during the same influenza season, even among elderly persons with weakened immune systems. Except for some children, only one dose of flu vaccine is recommended each season.

I) There was one study (published in 2012) that suggested that influenza vaccination might make people more susceptible to other respiratory infections. After that study was published, many experts looked into this issue further and conducted additional studies to see if the findings could be replicated. No other studies have found this effect. For example, this article in *Clinical Infectious Diseases* was published in 2013. It's not clear why this finding was detected in the one study, but the preponderance of evidence suggests that this is not a common or regular occurrence and that influenza vaccination does not, in fact, make people more susceptible to other respiratory infections.

J) CDC and the Advisory Committee on Immunization Practices (ACIP) recommend that flu vaccinations begin by the end of October, if possible. However, as long as flu viruses are circulating, it is not too late to get vaccinated, even in January or later. While seasonal flu outbreaks can happen as early as October, most of the time flu activity peaks between December and February, although activity can last as late as May. Since it takes about two weeks after vaccination for antibodies to develop in the body that protect against flu virus infection, it is best that people get vaccinated in time to be protected before flu viruses begin spreading in their community. Although immunity obtained from flu vaccination can vary by person, previously published studies suggest that immunity lasts through a full flu season for most people.

K) There is some evidence, however, that immunity may decline more quickly in older people. For older adults, two vaccine options are available. One of these options is a "high-dose" vaccine, which is designed specifically for people 65 and older.

2. Read the following statements. Decide to what extent you agree or disagree with each statement, and write your own pros or cons in the box, then set out your rational viewpoint and the reasons.

(1) Getting influenza vaccination helps to cut down the chances of getting sick. One important positive factor caused by influenza vaccination is the reduction of a chance for the disease.

(2) The allergic reactions of flu vaccination could be ignored, given to its positives.

Pros	Cons

VII. Outcome Sentence Analysis and Essay Writing

1. Sentence-structure analysis

Analyze the following sentences and draw a tree-structure.

(1) A pandemic is an epidemic of an infectious disease that has spread across a large region, for instance, multiple continents or worldwide, affecting a substantial number of people.

(2) Similarly, the number of recoveries may also be understated as tests are required before cases are officially recognized as recovered, and fatalities are sometimes attributed to other conditions.

(3) A disease of the large intestine and transmitted through contaminated water, cholera has haunted humanity for centuries.

(4) Research has indicated that each of the four historic influenza pandemics was preceded by a La Niña event — a change in global weather conditions associated with cool sea surface temperatures in the Pacific Ocean — which, some scientists speculate, may have altered the migratory patterns of birds, possibly increasing their interactions with domestic animals and enabling genetic reassortment and the rise of new pandemic strains of influenza viruses.

(5) The virus needs moisture and will dry out quickly if exposed to ultraviolet radiation or dry air, which may account for the prevalence of influenza during humid and darker winter weather.

2. **Essay writing**
   Influenced by the H1N1, many students have to ask for leave to have a rest. Write an e-mail to your friend Li Ming, telling him some useful tips during this period. You need to select 2 – 3 suggestions given by the following comic and write a 120-word e-mail to you friend.

Influenza A(H1N1)

How to Protect Yourself and Others

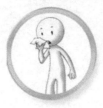 Cover your nose and mouth with a disposable tissue when coughing and sneezing

 Dispose of used tissues properly immediately after use

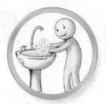 Regularly wash hands with soap and water

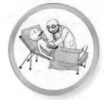 If you have flu-like symptoms, seek medical advice immediately

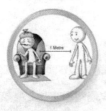 If you have flu-like symptoms, keep a distance of at least 1 meter from other people

 If you have flu-like symptoms, stay home from work, school or crowded places

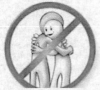 Avoid hugging, kissing and shaking hands when greeting

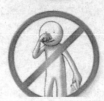 Avoid touching eyes, nose or mouth with unwashed hands

Unit 7
Psychology and Life

Read the web page. Then answer the questions orally.

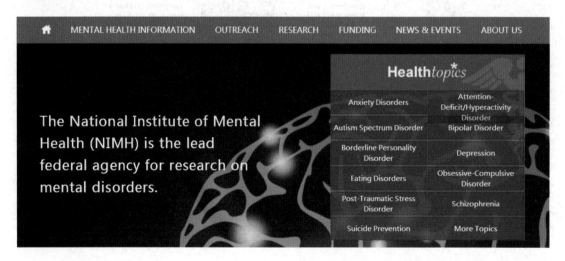

What is anxiety?

    Occasional anxiety is a normal part of life. Many people worry about things such as health, money, or family problems. But anxiety disorders involve more than temporary worry or fear. For people with an anxiety disorder, the anxiety does not go away and can get worse over time. The symptoms can interfere with daily activities such as job performance, schoolwork, and relationships.

There are several types of anxiety disorders, including generalized anxiety disorder, panic disorder, social anxiety disorder, and various phobia-related disorders.

Who gets depression?

Depression can affect people of all ages, races, ethnicities, and genders.

Women are diagnosed with depression more often than men, but men can also be depressed. Because men may be less likely to recognize, talk about, and seek help for their feelings or emotional problems, they are at greater risk of depression symptoms being undiagnosed or undertreated.

Statistics

Research shows that mental illnesses are common in the United States, affecting tens of millions of people each year. Estimates suggest that only half of people with mental illnesses receive treatment. The information on these pages includes currently available statistics on the prevalence and treatment of mental illnesses among the U.S. population. In addition, information is provided about possible consequences of mental illnesses, such as suicide and disability.

outreach [ˈaʊtriːtʃ]	*n.* the extending of services or assistance beyond current or usual linits 外展服务，扩大范围的服务
bipolar [baɪˈpəʊlə(r)]	*adj.* of or relating to manic depressive illness 双相型障碍的；躁狂抑郁性精神病的
borderline [ˈbɔːdəlaɪn]	*n.* a line that indicates a boundary 边界线
obsessive [əbˈsesɪv]	*adj.* characterized by or constituting an obsession 强迫性的
post-traumatic [ˌpəʊsttrɔːˈmætɪk]	*adj.* after a physical injury or wound to the body 受伤后的，创伤后的
schizophrenia [ˌskɪtsəˈfriːnɪə]	*n.* any of several psychotic disorders characterized by distortions of reality and disturbances of thought and language and withdrawal from social contact 精神分裂症

（1）What kind of information does NIMH offer from this web page?

_____

（2）What are the health conditions provided in this web page?

_____

（3）Why do men diagnosed with depression less often than women?

_____

（4）How many people with mental illnesses receive treatment ?

_____

II. Watching-in Knowledge about Psychology

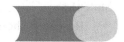

1. **View the video clips. Match the photos（A - D）to the dialogues（1 - 4）. Then answer the following questions.**

A.

B. questioning your decisions

C.

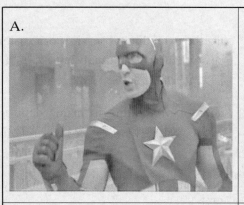

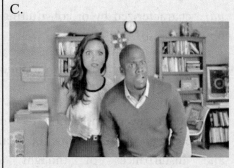

D.

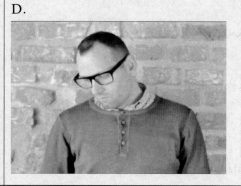

Video clip 1：_____   Video clip 2：_____

Video clip 3：_____   Video clip 4：_____

roadblock [ˈrəʊdblɒk]	*n.* any condition that makes it difficult to make progress or to achieve an objective 路障;障碍
accusatory [əˈkjuːzətərɪ]	*adj.* (formal) suggesting that you think sb has done sth wrong 谴责的;指责的;控告的
evoke [ɪˈvəʊk]	*v.* (formal) to bring a feeling, a memory or an image into your mind 引起,唤起(感情、记忆或形象)
lament [ləˈment]	*v.* (formal) to feel or express great sadness or disappointment about sb/sth 对……感到悲痛;痛惜;对……表示失望
flop [flɒp]	*v.* (informal) to be a complete failure 砸锅;完全失败
loathe [ləʊð]	*v.* to dislike sb/sth very much 极不喜欢;厌恶

(1) Where do our problems mostly come from?

_____

(2) Should we compare ourselves to others? Why and what should we do?

_____

(3) According to video 4, what is the most important thing?

_____

2. **View the video clips again. Fill in the blanks to complete the sentences which can help you get the gist of the content.**

(1)

If you had an amazing perfect 1) _____, that's great. But it also means that your problems come from somewhere else. And believe it or not, they mostly come from your mind. Just think about this, all that inner 2) _____ you have with yourself: questioning your decisions, 3) _____ what could have been if you've done something differently, trying to understand why someone acted in a certain way with you. What does all this change in your life? That's right. Nothing! These thoughts are absolutely 4) _____.

(2)

When we're not beating ourselves up, we're 1) _____ others for our problems. Of course, the people around us sometimes make mistakes that do affect us personally, but it's our job to deal with these 2) _____. If you've been hurt by someone, tell them how you feel, but choose your words 3) _____. Instead of saying "you betrayed me", a much better way to open a dialogue is to say "I feel betrayed". The first sentence is accusatory and will only cause the other person to go into 4) _____ mode and start arguing

When it comes to other people, sadly, we can't explain their behavior no matter how much we'd like to. They simply grew up in a different 5) _____ and have their own experiences that differ from ours. When you try to understand the 6) _____ behind someone else's actions, you face problems that you create yourself. And when it comes to beating yourself up for 7) _____, don't forget that you made that decision because you felt that it was right for you at that time in your life. The past is the past. Leave it there and 8) _____ it.

with you. The second phrase is closer to home and 5) _____ from the other person a sense of empathy and probably sincere 6) _____ for hurting you. You're not only honestly expressing your innermost 7) _____, you're also giving them a chance to do the same. And even if the situation can't be 8) _____, that's okay. It's in the past. You'll both still feel better after openly expressing your feelings.

(3)

Comparing yourself to others will get you nowhere. In your mind, you'll never 1) _____, and the same goes for everybody else, because we're all constantly comparing ourselves to others. Like we said before, everyone has their own 2) _____. They also have their own 3) _____, appearance, personal qualities and achievements. Who they are and what they have is different from you, and that's okay. That's what makes us all 4) _____. If you're 5) _____ by someone, that's great. Just try to have 6) _____ that are your own and not somebody else's. When we try to live another person's life, we 7) _____ our own. So learn more about yourself and create your own story. It's always better to be an 8) _____ than a bad copy.

(4)

The most important thing every single one of us should know how to do is to be our own 1) _____. You should be ready to admit 2) _____ and accept that you can't influence everything. Don't fall into the mental 3) _____ of thinking things over and over and lamenting all the time you 4) _____ working on something just to have it 5) _____. This sort of downward spiral of self-loathing and regret is literally 6) _____. You're the person you spend your whole life with. No matter how much everyone else 7) _____ you, if you don't like yourself, you'll still be miserable. Respect yourself, treat yourself right and expand your 8) _____. If you do that, you'll be unstoppable.

betray[bɪˈtreɪ]	v. to give information about sb/sth to an enemy 出卖；泄露（机密）
empathy[ˈempəθɪ]	n. the ability to understand another person's feelings, experience, etc. 同感；共鸣；同情
innermost[ˈɪnəməʊst]	adj. most private, personal and secret 内心深处的
lament[ləˈment]	v. to feel or express great sadness or disappointment about sb/sth 对…感到悲痛；痛惜；对…表示失望
self-loathing[ˌself ˈləʊðɪŋ]	adj. feel great dislike and disgust for oneself 自我讨厌的

III. Leading-in Defining Psychology

1. **View a video clip. Define the terms "psychology" using the following expressions.**

figures	underlying	motivation	grasp	insights	impact

experimentation	mechanisms	inform	interpret

Psychology is the science of the mind and human behavior. It aims to understand our (1)_____ mental functions, physiological and biological processes and internal (2)_____, things that determine our actions and behavior. Asking how and why we think, feel and act, it uses (3)_____ to investigate perception, intelligence, personality, cognition and (4)_____. Psychology lies at the heart of our efforts to (5)_____ what it is to be human. Its insights (6)_____ every other academic discipline. Studying the mind helps us to (7)_____ our own actions and understand why the (8)_____ of history made the decisions they did. It offers (9)_____ into the workings of the economy and makes it easier to chart the actions of the media and the (10)_____ of the law.

2. **Read the following passage and answer these questions.**

(1) What do you know about psychological studies?

_____

_____

(2) Who is Wilhelm Wundt? What is his work mainly about?

_____

_____

（3）Using the following terms to fill in the blanks in the last part of the passage.

Social	Industrial-organizational	Forensic	Cognitive	Abnormal
Clinical	Developmental	Personality	Biological	Comparative

Passage A

An Overview of Psychology

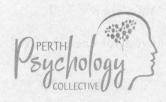

Psychology is a broad field that encompasses the study of human thought, behavior, development, personality, emotion, motivation, and more. Gaining a richer and deeper understanding of psychology can help people achieve insights into their own actions as well as a better understanding of others.

1. What Is Psychology?

Psychology is the study of the mind and behavior. Research in psychology seeks to understand and explain how people think, act, and feel. Psychologists strive to learn more about the many factors that can impact thought and behavior, ranging from biological influences to social pressures.

There's a lot of confusion out there about psychology. Unfortunately, such misconceptions about psychology abound in part thanks to stereotyped portrayals of psychologists in popular media as well as the diverse career paths of those holding psychology degrees.

According to some popular television programs and movies, psychologists are super-sleuths that can use their understanding of the human mind to solve crimes and predict a criminal's next move. Other traditional depictions present the psychologist as gray and wise, seated in a stately office lined with books, and listening to clients ramble on about their difficult childhoods.

So what is psychology really all about? There are psychologists who help solve crimes and there are plenty of professionals who help people deal with mental health issues. However, there are also psychologists who contribute to creating healthier workplaces. There are psychologists that design and implement public health programs. Other psychologists investigate topics such as airplane safety, computer design, and military life. No matter where psychologists work, their primary goals are to help describe, explain, predict, and influence human behavior.

Psychological studies are highly structured, beginning with a hypothesis that is then empirically tested. As psychology moved away from its philosophical roots, psychologists began to employ more and more scientific methods to study human behavior. Contemporary researchers use a variety of scientific techniques including experiments, correlational studies, and longitudinal research. As most people already realize, a large part of psychology is devoted to the diagnosis and treatment of mental health issues, but that's just the tip of the iceberg when it comes to applications of psychology. In addition to mental health, psychology can be applied to a variety of issues that impact health and daily life including well-being, ergonomics, motivation, productivity, and much more.

2. How Psychology Came to Be What It Is Today?

Early psychology evolved out of both philosophy and biology. Discussions of these two subjects date as far back as the early Greek thinkers, including Aristotle and Socrates. The word "psychology" itself is derived from the Greek word psyche, literally meaning "life" or "breath". Derived meanings of the word include "soul" or "self".

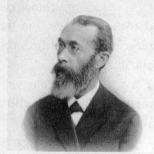

The emergence of psychology as a separate and independent field of study truly came about when Wilhelm Wundt established the first experimental psychology lab in Leipzig, Germany in 1879. Wundt's work was focused on describing the structures that compose the mind. This perspective relied heavily on the analysis of sensations and feelings through the use of introspection, an extremely subjective process. Wundt believed that properly trained individuals would be able to identify accurately the mental processes that accompanied feelings, sensations, and thoughts.

Wilhelm Wundt

Throughout psychology's history, various schools of thought have formed to explain the human mind and behavior. In some cases, certain schools of thought rose to dominate the field of psychology for a period of time. While these schools of thought are sometimes perceived as competing forces, each perspective has contributed to our understanding of psychology.

The following are some of the major schools of thought in psychology.

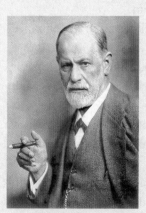

Wundt and Titchener's structuralism was the earliest school of thought, but others soon began to emerge. The early psychologist and philosopher William James became associated with a school of thought known as functionalism, which focused its attention on the purpose of human consciousness and behavior. Soon, these initial schools of thought gave way to several dominant and influential approaches to psychology. Sigmund Freud's psychoanalysis centered on the how the unconscious mind impacted human behavior. The behavioral school of thought turned away from looking at internal influences on behavior and sought to make

Sigmund Freud

psychology the study of observable behaviors. Later, the humanistic approach centered on the importance of personal growth and self-actualization. By the 1960s and 1970s, the cognitive revolution spurred the investigation of internal mental processes such as thinking, decision-making, language development, and memory.

3. There Are Many Different Specialty Areas in Psychology

Psychology is a broad and diverse field. Some different subfields and specialty areas have emerged. The following are some of the major areas of research and application within psychology:

_____ psychology is the study of abnormal behavior and psychopathology. This specialty area is focused on research and treatment of a variety of mental disorders and is linked to psychotherapy and clinical psychology.

_____ psychology, also known as biopsychology, studies how biological processes influence the mind and behavior. This area is closely linked to neuroscience and utilizes tools such as MRI and PET scans to look at brain injury or brain abnormalities.

_____ psychology is focused on the assessment, diagnosis, and treatment of mental disorders. It is also considered the single largest area of employment within psychology.

_____ psychology is the study of human thought processes and cognitions. Cognitive psychologists study topics such as attention, memory, perception, decision-making, problem-solving, and language acquisition.

_____ psychology is the branch of psychology concerned with the study of animal behavior. This type of research can lead to a deeper and broader understanding of human psychology.

_____ psychology is an area that looks at human growth and development over the lifespan. Theories often focus on the development of cognitive abilities, morality, social functioning, identity, and other life areas.

_____ psychology is an applied field focused on using psychological research and principles in the legal and criminal justice system.

_____ psychology is a field that uses psychological research to enhance work performance, and select employees.

_____ psychology focuses on understanding how personality develops as well as the patterns of thoughts, behaviors, and characteristics that make each individual unique.

_____ psychology focuses on understanding group behavior as well as how social influences shape individual behavior. Topics studied by social psychologists include attitudes, prejudice, conformity, and aggression.

While psychology may be a relatively young science it also has a tremendous amount of both depth and breadth. The assessment, diagnosis, and treatment of mental illness are central interests of psychology, but psychology encompasses much more than mental health. Today, psychologists seek to understand many different aspects of the human mind and behavior, adding new knowledge to our understanding of how people think as well as developing practical applications that have an important impact on everyday human lives.

misconception [ˌmɪskənˈsepʃən]	*n.* an incorrect conception 错误的概念；错误的想法
stereotyped [ˈsterɪəʊtaɪpt]	*adj.* lacking spontaneity or originality or individuality 墨守成规的；老旧的
sleuth [sluːθ]	*n.* a detective who follows a trail 侦探
empirically [ɪmˈpɪrɪkəlɪ]	*adv.* derived from experiment and observation rather than theory 以经验为主地
correlational [ˌkɒrəˈleɪʃənəl]	*adj.* relating to or employing correlation 相关的
longitudinal [ˌlɒndʒɪˈtjuːdɪnəl]	*adj.* concerning the development of sth over a period of time 纵观的
ergonomics [ˌɜːgəʊˈnɒmɪks]	*n.* the branch of engineering science in which biological science is used to study the relation between workers and their environments 工效学；人类工程学
introspection [ˌɪntrəʊˈspekʃən]	*n.* the contemplation of your own thoughts and desires and conduct 内省；反省
consciousness [ˈkɒnʃəsnɪs]	*n.* an alert cognitive state in which you are aware of yourself and your situation 意识；知觉；觉悟；感觉
psychoanalysis [ˌpsaɪkəʊəˈnæləsɪs]	*n.* medical treatment that involves talking to sb about their life, feelings, etc. in order to find out the causes of their problems 精神分析；心理分析
humanistic [ˌhjuːməˈnɪstɪk]	*adj.* pertaining to or concerned with the humanities 人文主义的；人道主义的
abnormal [æbˈnɔːməl]	*adj.* not normal; not typical or usual or regular or conforming to a norm 反常的，不规则的；变态的
psychopathology [ˌpsaɪkəʊpəˈθɒlədʒɪ]	*n.* the study of the origin, development, and manifestations of mental or behavioral disorders 精神病理学
forensic [fəˈrensɪk]	*adj.* of, relating to, or used in courts of law or public debate or argument 法院的；辩论的；适于法庭的

3. Match each of the terms listed below with the numbered definition. Write the letter in the space provided.

A. humanistic	E. introspection	I. stereotyped
B. unconscious	F. cognitive	J. hypothesis
C. psychopathology	G. derived	K. self-actualization
D. psychoanalysis	H. encompass	L. behaviorism

（1） _____ : to include in scope; to include as part of something broader

（2） _____ : lacking spontaneity or originality or individuality

（3） _____ : lacking awareness and the capacity for sensory perception as if asleep or dead

（4） _____ : of or pertaining to a philosophy asserting human dignity and man's capacity for fulfillment through reason and scientific method and often rejecting religion

（5） _____ : a proposal intended to explain certain facts or observations; a tentative theory about the natural world

（6） _____ : the scientific study of mental disorders

（7） _____ : of or being or relating to or involving cognition

（8） _____ : the contemplation of your own thoughts and desires and conduct

（9） _____ : a set of techniques for exploring underlying motives and a method of treating various mental disorders

（10） _____ : formed or developed from something else; not original

（11） _____ : the motive to realize one's full potential

（12） _____ : the belief held by some psychologists that the only valid method of studying the psychology of people or animals is to observe how they behave

IV. Critical Reading — Further Reading on Psychology

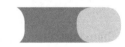

1. **An Overview of Humanistic Psychology**

   Read the following passage and complete the exercises that follow.

   A. Fill in the blanks to complete the table.

（1）Definition and key points
Humanistic psychology, often known as 1) _____ , is a perspective that stresses looking at the whole individual and emphasizes concepts such as 2) _____ , 3) _____ , and 4) _____ .
（2）The development of humanistic psychology
In the late 1950s, 5) _____ appeared, primarily in response to the 6) _____ and 7) _____ .

In 1957 and 1958, Abraham Maslow and other psychologists discussed developing a professional organization devoted to a more 8) _____ to psychology.

In 1961, the American Association for Humanistic Psychology, which in 1971 became an APA 9) _____, was formed.

In 1962, Maslow described humanistic psychology as the 10) _____ in psychology in his book.

(3) Strengths and criticisms

Strengths: It emphasizes the role of 11) _____; taking 12) _____ into account; making therapy more 13) _____ for normal, healthy individuals.

Criticisms: It is too 14) _____; observations are 15) _____; no 16) _____ way to measure or quantify these qualities.

B. Judge whether the following statements are true (T) or false (F).

_____ (1) Behaviorism was focused on understanding the unconscious motivations that drive behavior.

_____ (2) The belief that people are good by nature is the very fundamental concept of humanism.

_____ (3) Psychoanalysis was criticized for its strong emphasis on unconscious and instinctive forces and for being deterministic.

_____ (4) Humanistic psychology assumes that self-actualization is natural.

_____ (5) Humanistic psychology concentrates solely on our internal thoughts and desires.

Passage B

An Overview of Humanistic Psychology

Humanistic psychology, often referred to as humanism, is a perspective that emphasizes looking at the whole individual and stresses concepts such as free will, self-efficacy, and self-actualization. It was a reaction to the psychoanalysis and behaviorism that dominated psychology at the time. Psychoanalysis was focused on understanding the unconscious motivations that drive behavior while behaviorism studied the conditioning processes that produce behavior. Humanist thinkers felt that both 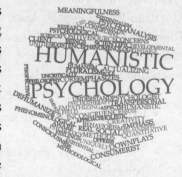 psychoanalysis and behaviorism were too pessimistic, either focusing on the most tragic of emotions or failing to take into account the role of personal choice.

However, it is not necessary to think of these three schools of thought as competing elements. Each branch of psychology has contributed to our understanding of the human mind and behavior. Humanistic psychology added yet another dimension that takes a more holistic view of the individual.

Humanism is grounded in the belief that people are innately good. This type of psychology holds that morality, ethical values, and good intentions are the driving forces of behavior, while adverse social or psychological experiences can be attributed to deviations from natural tendencies. Humanism incorporates a variety of therapeutic techniques, including Rogerian (person-centered) therapy, and often emphasizes a goal of self-actualization.

The Development of Humanistic Psychology

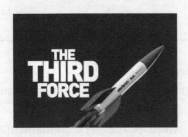

Humanism arose in the late 1950s as a "third force" in psychology, primarily in response to what some psychologists viewed as significant limitations in the behaviorist and psychoanalytic schools of thought. Behaviorism was often criticized for lacking focus on human consciousness and personality and for being deterministic, mechanistic, and over-reliant on animal studies. Psychoanalysis was rejected for its strong emphasis on unconscious and instinctive forces and for being deterministic, as well.

In 1957 and 1958, Abraham Maslow and Clark Moustakas met with psychologists who shared their goal of establishing a professional association that emphasized a more positive and humanistic approach. The discussions revolved around the topics they believed would become the core tenets of this new approach to psychology: self-actualization, creativity, health, individuality, intrinsic nature, self, being, becoming, and meaning.

After receiving sponsorship, the American Association for Humanistic Psychology was founded in 1961 and by 1971, humanistic psychology became an American Psychological Association (APA) division. In 1962, Maslow published *Toward a Psychology of Being*, in which he described humanistic psychology as the "third force" in psychology. The first and second forces were behaviorism and psychoanalysis respectively.

Some fundamental assumptions of humanistic psychology include:

- Experiencing (thinking, sensing, perceiving, feeling, remembering, and so on) is central.
- The subjective experience of the individual is the primary indicator of behavior.
- An accurate understanding of human behavior cannot be achieved by studying animals.
- Free will exists, and individuals should take personal responsibility for self-growth and fulfillment. Not all behavior is determined.
- Self-actualization (the need for a person to reach maximum potential) is natural.

- People are inherently good and will experience growth if provided with suitable conditions，especially during childhood.
- Each person and each experience is unique，so psychologists should treat each case individually，rather than rely on averages from group studies.

Strengths and Criticisms of Humanistic Psychology

One of the major strengths of humanistic psychology is that it emphasizes the role of the individual. This school of psychology gives people more credit in controlling and determining their state of mental health. It also takes environmental influences into account. Rather than focusing solely on our internal thoughts and desires，humanistic psychology also credits the environment's influence on our experiences.

Humanistic psychology helped remove some of the stigma attached to therapy and made it more acceptable for normal，healthy individuals to explore their abilities and potential through therapy.

While humanistic psychology continues to influence therapy，education，healthcare，and other areas，it has not been without some criticism. Humanistic psychology is often seen as too subjective；the importance of individual experience makes it difficult to objectively study and measure humanistic phenomena. How can we objectively tell if someone is self-actualized? The answer，of course，is that we cannot. We can only rely upon the individual's own assessment of their experience. Another major criticism is that observations are unverifiable；there is no accurate way to measure or quantify these qualities.

holistic [həʊˈlɪstɪk]	*adj*. emphasizing the organic or functional relation between parts and the whole 整体的；全盘的
therapeutic [ˌθerəˈpjuːtɪk]	*adj*. tending to cure or restore to health 治疗的；治疗学的；有益于健康的
intrinsic [ɪnˈtrɪnsɪk]	*adj*. belonging to a thing by its very nature 本质的；固有的
unverifiable [ˌʌnˈverɪfaɪəbl]	*adj*. not objective or easily verified 无法核实的；无法检验的

2. **Q & A of** *Basic Construction Standards for Students' Mental Health Education in General Institutions of Higher Learning*（*for Trial Implementation*）
   Read the following passage to complete the note-taking table，and then check your understanding.

Colleges and universities integrate mental health education into the school talent training system.	We should (1)_____ a special leading body, (2)_____ by school leaders responsible for the mental health education involving conselling institutions, student work department ...
The responsibilities of the three levels of mental health education	The colleges and universities should have the institutions (3)_____ for college students' (4)_____ education and counseling, into the (5)_____ and political education system of school, the specific organization and (6)_____ work of students' psychological health education school.
The construction of college students' mental health education system	First, colleges and universities should (7)_____ the role of classroom teaching in college students' (8)_____ health education, and establish or perfect the corresponding curriculum system according to the needs of psychological health education. Second, colleges and universities should (9)_____ the laws and characteristics of students' psychological development, scientifically (10)_____ the content of the course of psychological health education for college students, and effectively (11)_____ the teaching methods of education.

Passage C

Q & A of *Basic Construction Standards for Students' Mental Health Education in General Institutions of Higher Learning* (*for Trial Implementation*)

For the further implementation of the spirit of the National Education Conference, the education plan and the National Forum to Strengthen and Improve College Students' Ideological and Political Education, and the "CPC Central Committee and State Council on Further Strengthening and Improving Ideological and Political Education" (No. 16, 2004), Basic Construction Standards for Students' Mental Health Education in General Institutions of Higher Learning (for Trial Implementation) is formulated to promote scientific construction of college students' psychological health education. This standard shall be put into effect on the date of issuance. It shall be applicable to ordinary institutions of higher learning, and shall serve as a frame of reference to other types of colleges and universities.

Here are the questions and answers by a student and a teacher.

Student: Why should we construct the system of college students' psychological health education?

Teacher: Under the new situation, strengthening and improving college students' mental health education is an important way to implement the spirit of the National Education Conference and the outline of the national medium and long-term education reform and development Plan (2010 - 2020). It is also a measure of the comprehensive education policy to cultivate innovative talents. The construction of talent team is an important task to carry out the Party's policy, promote the reform of higher education, strengthen and improve the ideological and political education of college students.

Student: How is the system and mechanism of College Students' Psychological Health Education constructed?

Teacher: 1. Colleges and universities should integrate the mental health education into the school talent training system.

2. Colleges and universities should have a sound network of three level mental health education involving schools, colleges and universities and students' classes, and all departments at all levels should have a clear division of responsibilities and coordination mechanism.

3. Universities should, according to the actual situation, study and formulate the views or implementation methods of psychological health education for college students. The mechanism of assessment, rewards and penalties should be established and the annual work plan shall be worked out.

4. Universities should concentrate on the mental health education and counseling agencies with standardized management, psychological crisis prevention and intervention, psychological counseling, mental health education curriculum teaching process, mental health education practitioners up to occupation moral standards, should establish and improve various rules and regulations.

Student: How should colleges and universities integrate the mental health education into the school talent training system?

Teacher: We should set up a special leading body, designated by school leaders responsible for the mental health education involving conselling institutions, student work department, propaganda department, administration department, personnel department, financial department, security department and the logistics service department, University Hospital and the hospital (or department), Graduate School and related disciplines, teaching and research units responsible for human members. The leading body is responsible for research and develop students' mental health education planning and related systems, the overall leadership of the mental health education of College students. The Standing Committee of the Party Commission or the president's office shall regularly hear special reports, study and deploy the tasks, and solve the existing problems.

Student: What are the responsibilities of the three levels of mental health education?

Teacher: The colleges and universities should have the institutions responsible for college students' mental health education and counseling, into the ideological and political education system of school, the specific organization and coordination work of students' psychological health education school; College (Department) shall arrange part-time teachers responsible for the implementation of mental health education;

Organize the students to the class committee, Party branch and other student organizations to actively assist the instructors and graduate instructors to carry out mental health education work.

Student: How do colleges and universities carry out the construction of teachers' team for college students' Psychological Health Education?

Teacher: 1. Colleges and universities should build a team of teachers with mental health education and psychological counseling with the full-time teachers as the backbone, and the students who are both specialized and integrated, relatively stable and of high quality.

2. Colleges and universities should incorporate the construction of teachers' mental health education staff into the overall construction of teachers' team, and strengthen the selection, equipment, training and management.

3. Colleges and universities should pay attention to the mental health education of college students, and the specialized training of part-time teachers.

4. All faculty and staff in colleges and universities have the responsibility to educate and guide students' healthy growth, and should focus on building a harmonious and good teacher-student relationship, and strengthen the awareness of full participation of College Students' psychological health education.

Student: what do you mean that colleges and universities should incorporate the construction of teachers' mental health education staff into the overall construction of teachers' team?

Teacher: Teachers engaged in mental health education for college students, especially those who are directly engaged in psychological counseling, should have relevant academic qualifications and professional qualifications to engage in mental health education for college students. Full-time teachers should be included in the ranks of the ideological and political education teachers, and schools with educational, psychological, medical and other teaching and research institutions can also be included in the corresponding professional sequence. The part-time teachers should carry out psychological counseling and consultation activities, and the corresponding workload should be calculated.

Student: How to construct College Students' mental health education system?

Teacher: First, colleges and universities should give full play to the role of classroom teaching in college students' psychological health education, and establish or perfect the corresponding curriculum system according to the needs of psychological health education. Schools should set up compulsory or elective courses, giving appropriate credit guarantee to the students who have generally received psychological health education.

Second, colleges and universities should take full account of the laws and characteristics of students' psychological development, scientifically regulate the content of the course of psychological health education for college students, and effectively improve the teaching methods of education. There should be special teaching outline or basic teaching requirements. Teaching content design should combine theory and practice, and be easily accessible to students. We should improve the effect of classroom teaching by means of case study, experience activity and behavior training, and improve teaching quality through teaching research and reform.

Student：How about the construction of College Students' psychological health education system?

Teacher：First，colleges and universities should carry out mental health education activities for all students，innovate the forms of mental health education activities，expand the ways of mental health education，and actively create a good mental health education atmosphere.

Second，the construction of mental health education and counseling field should accord with the characteristics and requirements of College Students' mental health education，and can meet the needs of students' education and counselling. The mental health education and counselling area includes reservation waiting room，individual counselling room，group counseling room，psychological evaluation room and so on.

Third，colleges and universities should provide psychological health education and institutions with necessary office equipment，commonly used psychological measurement tools，statistical analysis software and mental health books and other mental health education products.

ideological [ˌaɪdɪəʊˈlɒdʒɪkəl]	*adj*. concerned with or suggestive of ideas 思想体系的；意识形态的
issuance [ˈɪʃjuːəns]	*n*. the act of providing an item for general use or for official purposes（usually in quantity）发布，发行
deploy [dɪˈplɔɪ]	*v*. to use sth effectively 有效地利用；调动

3. **Lexical chunks and sentence rewriting.**

   A. **Substitute the underline part with the words or expressions you have learned.**

   （1）Psychologists strive to learn more about the many factors that can ...（Passage A）

   Answer：

   Psychologists _____ learn more about the many factors that can ...

   （2）Psychological studies are highly structured，beginning with a hypothesis that ...（Passage A）

   Answer：

   Psychological studies are highly structured，_____ a hypothesis that ...

   （3）Early psychology evolved out of both philosophy and biology.（Passage A）

   Answer：

   Early psychology _____ both philosophy and biology.

   （4）... the cognitive revolution spurred the investigation of internal mental processes ...（Passage A）

   Answer：

... the cognitive revolution _____ the investigation of internal mental processes ...

（5）Each branch of psychology has <u>contributed to</u> our understanding of the human mind and behavior. （Passage B）

Answer：

Each branch of psychology has _____ our understanding of the human mind and behavior.

（6）Humanism <u>incorporates</u> a variety of therapeutic techniques，including ... （Passage B）

Answer：

Humanism _____ a variety of therapeutic techniques，including ...

（7）Humanism <u>arose</u> in the late 1950s as a "third force" in psychology，<u>primarily in</u> ...（Passage B）

Answer：

Humanism _____ in the late 1950s as a "third force" in psychology，_____ in ...

（8）Basic construction standards for students' mental health education in general institutions of higher learning（for Trial Implementation）is <u>formulated</u> to promote scientific construction of college students' psychological health education. （Passage C）

Answer：

Basic construction standards for students' mental health education in general institutions of higher learning（for Trial Implementation）is _____ to promote scientific construction of college students' psychological health education. （Passage C）

B. Rewrite the following sentences using the academic expressions you have learned in the articles.

（1）As most people already realize，a large part of psychology is dedicated to the diagnosis and treatment of mental health issues，but that's just the tip of the iceberg when it comes to applications of psychology.

Lexical chunks： _____

Sentence rewriting： _____

（2）Discussions of these two subjects go back as far as the early Greek thinkers，including Aristotle and Socrates.

Lexical chunks： _____

Sentence rewriting： _____

（3）Each branch of psychology makes contribution to our understanding of the human mind and behavior.

Lexical chunks： _____

Sentence rewriting： _____

(4) Humanism is earthed in the belief that people are innately good.

Lexical chunks: _____

Sentence rewriting: _____

(5) The part-time teachers should perform psychological counseling and consultation activities, and the corresponding workload should be calculated.

Lexical chunks: _____

Sentence rewriting: _____

4. **Bilingual translation**

Put the following into Chinese or vice versa.

A. English-Chinese translation

Learn the following useful expressions by translating the sentences selected from the passages.

(1) insights into 深刻理解,洞察

Excerpt:

Gaining a richer and deeper understanding of psychology can help people achieve insights into their own actions as well as a better understanding of others.

Translation:

_____

_____

(2) the tip of the iceberg 冰山一角;很小的一部分

Excerpt:

As most people already realize, a large part of psychology is devoted to the diagnosis and treatment of mental health issues, but that's just the tip of the iceberg when it comes to applications for psychology.

Translation:

_____

_____

(3) gave way to 给……让路;被……取代

Excerpt:

Soon, these initial schools of thought gave way to several dominant and influential approaches to psychology.

Translation:

_____

_____

(4) be referred to as 被称为

Excerpt:

Humanistic psychology, also often referred to as humanism, emerged during the 1950s as a reaction to the psychoanalysis and behaviorism that dominated psychology at the time.

Translation：

_____

_____

（5）be grounded in　以……为基础，以……为根据

Excerpt：

Humanism is grounded in the belief that people are innately good.

Translation：

_____

_____

（6）give full play to 充分发挥

Excerpt：

First，colleges and universities should give full play to the role of classroom teaching in college students' psychological health education，and establish or perfect the corresponding curriculum system according to the needs of psychological health education.

Translation：

_____

_____

B. Chinese-English translation

Put the Chinese paragraph into English.

《通知》强调，通过完善"学校、部门、班级、宿舍/个人"四级预警体系，建立健全日常预警体系。学校应该注意他们的学生是否遭受了毁灭性的事故或挫折，或者是否有明显的异常表现。学校应及时收集学生是否面临早期心理创伤、重大家庭变化或家庭关系紧张等困难的信息，并积极寻求学生家庭成员或相关方的建设性支持。中小学教师应与学生家长经常进行深入的沟通，互相提高心理辅导能力。高校应加强心理咨询平台建设，建立心理发展咨询室，开展个体心理咨询或团体心理咨询。同时，高校应配备专职心理健康导师，至少为4 000名学生配备一名导师。具体而言，每所学校至少应有两名心理健康教师，并将心理健康教育列为必修课程。

_____

_____

_____

_____

_____

_____

_____

_____

_____

_____

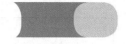

V. Speaking-out | The Four Major Specific Phobia Catergories

1. Read and say.

Look at the pictures and read the information on them. Work in pairs to share your understanding of them. Mark down the interesting ideas of your classmates.

Speaking skills:
Read the pictures and tell the story. Here are the steps:
(1) Choose one of the specific phobia categories and describe it. Describe what you see and create sentences.
(2) Check the facts in the Internet and write down the interesting points and new ideas of your classmates.
(3) Create 10 - 15 sentences relating to the the symtoms, the causes, the diagnosis and treatment of the specific phobia category based on your understanding. Be as creative and imaginative as you can. Attention should be paid to both explicit and implicit meaning.
(4) Read the sentences aloud and then start correcting the sentences on your own.

More useful expressions:	
fear/horror/terror	a group of anxiety symptoms
long lasting/unreasonable/irrational	exposure to the specific object
intensive nervousness	a full-scale anxiety attack
traumatic experience or learned reaction	potentially dangerous situation
respond to the objects with fear	psychiatric history
reported symptoms	cognitive behavior therapy
relaxation techniques	severe anxiety disorder
excessive fear of a situation	dizziness/trembling/increased heart rate
breathlessness	preoccupation with the feared object
imagined illnesses or imminent death	a sense of endangerment

pictures	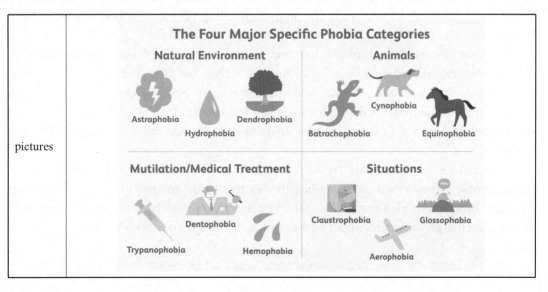

points	_____
	_____
	_____
	_____
	_____
	_____
	_____
	_____
	_____
	_____
	_____

2. Watch and act.

Watch a video clip. Fill in the blanks and then act it out in class.

I am a health psychologist, and my (1)_____ is to help people be happier and healthier. But I (2)_____ that something I've been teaching for the last 10 years is doing more harm than good, and it has to do with stress. For years, I've been telling people: Stress makes you sick. It increases the risk of everything from the common cold to (3)_____. Basically, I've turned stress into the (4)_____. But I have changed my mind about stress, and today, I want to change yours.

Let me start with the study that made me (5)_____ my whole approach to stress. This study (6)_____ 30,000 adults in the United States for eight years, and they started by asking people, "How much stress did you experienced in the last year?" They also asked, "Do you believe that stress is harmful for your health?" And then they used public (7)_____ to find out who died.

Okay. Some bad news first. People who experienced a lot of stress in the previous year had a 43 percent (8)_____ risk of dying. But that was only true for the people who also believed that stress is harmful for your health. People who experienced a lot of stress but did not view stress as harmful were no more likely to die. In fact, they had the (9)_____ of dying of anyone in the study, including people who had relatively little stress.

Now the researchers estimated that over the eight years they were tracking deaths, 182,000 Americans died (10)_____, not from stress, but from the (11)_____ that stress is bad for you. That is over 20,000 deaths a year. Now, if that (12)_____ is correct, that would make believing stress is bad for you the 15th largest (13)_____ in the United States last year, killing more people than skin cancer, HIV/AIDS and homicide.

You can see why this study freaks me out. Here I've been spending so much energy telling people stress is bad for your health. So this study got me (14)_____: Can changing how you think about stress make you healthier? And here the science says yes. When you change your mind about stress, you can change your body's (15)_____ to stress.

Ten Ways Psychology Can Help You Live a Better Life

1. Read the following passage with ten statements attached to it. Each statement contains information given in one of the paragraphs. Identify the paragraph from which the information is derived. You may choose a paragraph more than once. Each paragraph is marked with a letter.

_____ (1) Nonverbal signals is very important in our interpersonal communications.

_____ (2) Eliminating distractions helps to increase one's memory power.

_____ (3) Setting clear goals that are directly related to the task can increase your motivational level.

_____ (4) Psychology can be used in many ways for its applied and theoretical nature.

_____ (5) Not everyone is a born leader.

_____ (6) Test-taking is probably a better memory aid than studying.

_____ (7) Cognitive psychologists have provided a lot of information about decision making.

_____ (8) Emotional intelligence can be improved by seeing situations from the perspective of others.

_____ (9) In order to become more productive, one should focus on the task at hand and eliminate distractions.

_____ (10) Behavior economics has produced some important findings that one can use to make wiser financial decision.

A) How can psychology apply to your everyday life? Do you think that psychology is just for students, academics, and therapists? Then think again. Because psychology is both an applied and a theoretical subject, it can be utilized in a number of ways. While research studies aren't exactly light reading material for the average person, the results of these experiments and studies can have significant applications in daily life. The following are some of the top ten practical uses for psychology in everyday life.

1. Get motivated.

B) Whether your goal is to quit smoking, lose weight, or learn a new language, some lessons from psychology offer tips for getting motivated. To increase your motivational levels when approaching a task, utilize some of the following tips derived from research in cognitive and educational psychology:

- Introduce new or novel elements to keep your interest high.
- Vary the sequence to help stave off boredom.
- Learn new things that build on your existing knowledge.
- Set clear goals that are directly related to the task.
- Reward yourself for a job well done.

2. Improve your leadership skills.

C) It doesn't matter if you're an office manager or a volunteer at a local youth group, having good leadership skills will probably be essential at some point in your life. Not everyone is a born leader, but a few simple tips gleaned from psychological research can help you improve your leadership skills. One of the most famous studies on this topic looked at three distinct leadership styles. Based on the findings of this study and subsequent research, practice some of the following when you are in a leadership position:

- Offer clear guidance, but allow group members to voice opinions.
- Talk about possible solutions to problems with members of the group.
- Focus on stimulating ideas and be willing to reward creativity.

3. Become a better communicator.

D) Communication involves much more than how you speak or write. Research suggests that nonverbal signals make up a huge portion of our interpersonal communications. To communicate your message effectively, you need to learn how to express yourself nonverbally and to read the nonverbal cues of those around you. A few key strategies include the following:

- Use good eye contact.
- Start noticing nonverbal signals in others.
- Learn to use your tone of voice to reinforce your message.

4. Learn to better understand others.

E) Much like nonverbal communication, your ability to understand your emotions and the emotions of those around you plays an important role in your relationships and professional life. The term "emotional intelligence" refers to your ability to understand both your own emotions as well as those of other people. Your emotional intelligence quotient is a measure of this ability. According to psychologist Daniel Goleman, your EQ may actually be more important than your IQ. What can you do to become more emotionally intelligent? Consider some of the following strategies:

- Carefully assess your own emotional reactions.
- Record your experience and emotions in a journal.
- Try to see situations from the perspective of another person.

5. Make more accurate decisions.

F) Research in cognitive psychology has provided a wealth of information about decisionmaking. By applying these strategies to your life, you can learn to make wiser choices. The next time you need to make a big decision, try using some of the following techniques:

- Try using the "six thinking hats" approach by looking at the situation from multiple points of view, including rational, emotional, intuitive, creative, positive, and negative perspectives.
- Consider the potential costs and benefits of a decision.
- Employ a grid analysis technique that gives a score for how a particular decision will satisfy specific requirements you may have.

6. Improve your memory.

G) Have you ever wondered why you can remember exact details of childhood events yet forget the name of the new client you met yesterday? Research on how we form new memories as well as how and why we forget has led to a number of findings that can be applied directly in your daily life. What are some ways you can increase your memory power?

- Focus on the information.
- Rehearse what you have learned.
- Eliminate distractions.

7. Make wiser financial decisions.

H) Nobel Prize-winning psychologist Daniel Kahneman and his colleague Amos Tversky conducted a series of studies that looked at how people manage uncertainty and risk when making decisions. Subsequent research in this area known as behavior economics has yielded some key findings that you can use to make wiser money management choices. One study found that workers could more than triple their savings by utilizing some of the following strategies：

- Don't procrastinate. Start investing in savings now.
- Commit in advance to devote portions of your future earnings to your retirement savings.
- Try to be aware of personal biases that may lead to poor money choices.

8. Get better grades.

I) The next time you're tempted to complain about pop quizzes, midterms, or final exams, consider that research has demonstrated that taking tests actually helps you better remember what you've learned, even if it wasn't covered on the test. Another study found that repeated test-taking may be a better memory aid than studying. Students who were tested repeatedly were able to recall 61 percent of the material while those in the study group recalled only 40 percent. How can you apply these findings to your own life? When trying to learn new information, self-test frequently in order to cement what you have learned into your memory.

9. Become more productive.

J) Sometimes it seems like there are thousands of books, blogs, and magazine articles telling us how to get more done in a day, but how much of this advice is founded on actual research? For example, think about the number of times you have heard that multitasking can help you become more productive. In reality, research has found that trying to perform more than one task at the same time seriously impairs speed, accuracy, and productivity. So what lessons from psychology can you use to increase your productivity? Consider some of the following：

- Avoid multitasking when working on complex or dangerous tasks.
- Focus on the task at hand.
- Eliminate distractions.

10. Be healthier.

K) Psychology can also be a useful tool for improving your overall health. From ways to encourage exercise and better nutrition to new treatments for depression, the field of health psychology offers a wealth of beneficial strategies that can help you to be healthier and happier. Some examples that you can apply directly to your own life:

- Studies have shown that both sunlight and artificial light can reduce the symptoms of seasonal affective disorder.

- Research has demonstrated that exercise can contribute to greater psychological well-being.

- Studies have found that helping people understand the risks of unhealthy behaviors can lead to healthier choices.

2. Read the following statements. Decide to what extent you agree or disagree with each statement, and write your own pros or cons in the box, then set out your rational viewpoints and the reasons.

（1）The breadth and diversity of psychology can be seen by looking at some of its best-known thinkers.

（2）Learning would be exceedingly laborious, not to mention hazardous, if people had to rely solely on the effects of their own actions to inform them what to do.

Pros	Cons

VII. Outcome — Sentence Analysis and Essay Writing

1. Sentence-structure analysis

Analyze the following sentences and draw a tree-structure.

(1) Unfortunately, such misconceptions about psychology abound in part thanks to stereotyped portrayals of psychologists in popular media as well as the diverse career paths of those holding psychology degrees.

(2) Today, psychologists seek to understand many different aspects of the human mind and behavior, adding new knowledge to our understanding of how people think as well as developing practical applications that have an important impact on everyday human lives.

(3) In 1957 and 1958, Abraham Maslow and Clark Moustakas met with psychologists who shared their goal of establishing a professional association that emphasized a more positive and humanistic approach.

2. Essay writing

Write an essay on Psychology and Life. Search for relevant information via the Internet or books in the library. The following outline is for your reference.

Outline:

(1) What is psychology?

(2) What are the main psychological problems for college students nowadays?

(3) How does psychological knowledge help in your life?

_____
_____
_____
_____
_____
_____
_____
_____
_____
_____

Unit 8
Drug Safety

I. Info-storm   Web News on Medication Safety

Read the web page. Then answer the questions orally.

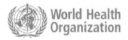
World Health
Organization

The Third WHO Global Patient Safety Challenge: Medication Without Harm

Unsafe medication practices and medication errors are a leading cause of injury and avoidable harm in healthcare systems across the world. Globally, the cost associated with medication errors has been estimated at $42 billion USD annually. Errors can occur at different stages of the medication use process. Medication errors occur when weak medication systems and/or human factors such as fatigue, poor environmental conditions or staff shortages affect prescribing, transcribing, dispensing, administration and monitoring practices, which can then result in severe harm, disability and even death. Multiple interventions to address the frequency and impact of medication errors have already been developed, yet their implementation is varied. A wide mobilization of stakeholders supporting sustained actions is required. In response to this, WHO has identified "Medication Without Harm" as the theme for the Third Global Patient Safety Challenge.

transcribe [træn'skraɪb]	v. to write, type, or print out fully from speech, notes, etc. 记录
dispense [dɪ'spens]	v. to prepare medicines and give them to people 配药
administration [ədˌmɪnɪ'streɪʃən]	n. the act of giving a drug to sb 给药

208

(1) What is a leading cause of injury and avoidable harm in healthcare systems?

_____

(2) Why do medication errors occur?

_____

(3) What are the results of medication errors?

_____

(4) What's the theme for the Third Global Patient Safety Challenge?

_____

II. Watching-in Broke Girls' Drug Test

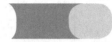

1. View the video clips. Match the photos (A – D) to the video clips (1 – 4). Then answer the following questions.

A.

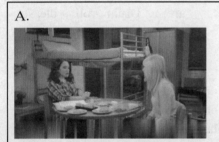

B.

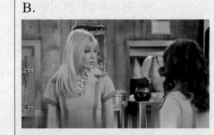

C.

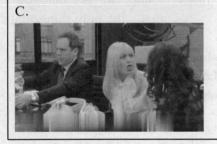

D.

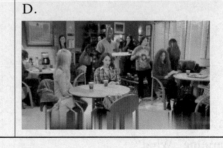

Video clip 1: _____   Video clip 2: _____
Video clip 3: _____   Video clip 4: _____

(1) Why do the broke girls go to the drug test?

_____

(2) What are the side effects mentioned by the nurse? List at least five.

_____

(3) What side effect does Caroline have after taking the drug?

_____

（4）Why does the prosecutor ask Leo to take Caroline to the rehab?

_____

2. View the video clips again. Fill in the blanks to complete the sentences which can help you get the gist of the content.

(1)	(2)
Caroline：Max，I am not doing a drug 1)_____. Besides，it's not enough money anyway. **Max**：No，but after I put in my $500，plus we take $100 from the cupcake 2)_____. **Caroline**：You would do that for me? You know，I always thought we'd have to use the cupcake money to get us out of a legal problem. I just thought it'd be for you. **Max**：Me too! Welcome 3)_____，drug buddy.	**Toby**：Now，since most of you have done this before，I'll make it quick. Half of you will get a 1)_____. The other half will testing on a new drug called Gladiva. And no，that's not my stage name down at the clubs. Okay，possible side effects may occur over the next 24 to 48 hours. They are... Drum roll，please... Headaches，2)_____，flatulence，tongue-swelling，3)_____ thoughts... **Caroline**：I'm having some right now. **Toby**：ITW... **Max**：Inability to walk. **Caroline**：I hope we get that 'cause that's the only thing that's gonna keep me here. **Toby**：And RU... **Max**：Relentless urination. **Toby**：4)_____，seizures.
(3)	(4)
Caroline：What? **Max**：Mm，it's probably nothing，but she might be 1)_____ RU. **Caroline**：What's that again? **Max**：Relentless 2)_____. **Caroline**：She just said she had to 3)_____. **Max**：Yeah，that's relentless. **Caroline**：Are you okay?	**Caroline**：No，I had no knowledge of that transaction. （not clear） **Lawyer**：Could you repeat that? **Max**：Ruh-roh. You're having a side effect! Tongue 1)_____. TS! ··· **Leo**：Uh，counselor，give us one second. What is going on?

Unknown：Yeah. **Max**："RU" sure?	**Caroline**：We took drugs. **Leo**：Did she just say 'we took drugs'? **Max**：Very good，Leo. You must play charades. Look，we did a drug trial to get money for this. **Lawyer**：What's the holdup, counselor? **Max**：Just give her some water. I had this once. It goes away in an hour. **Caroline**：You said you never had any side effects! **Max**：Oh，please. I died once. I just didn't want to 2)_____ you.

relentless [rɪˈlentlɪs]　　*adj*. not stopping or getting less strong 不停的；持续强烈的

urination [ˌjʊərɪˈneɪʃən]　　*n*. the bodily process of discharging waste matter 排尿

transaction [trænˈzækʃən]　　*n*. the action or process of buying or selling sth 交易

III. Leading-in　Drug Mechanism

1. **View a video clip and fill in the blanks. Then describe how pills work on human body.**

　　Most people will take a pill，receive an (1) _____ ，or otherwise take some kind of medicine during their lives，but most of us don't know anything about how these (2) _____ actually work. How can various (3) _____ impact the way we physically feel，think，and even behave? For the most part，this depends on how a drug (4) _____ the communication between cells in the brain. There are a number of different ways that can happen. But before it gets into the brain，any drug must first reach the bloodstream on a journey that can take anywhere from seconds to hours，depending on factors like how it's (5) _____ . The slowest method is to take a drug orally because it must be absorbed by our digestive system before it takes effect. Inhaling a drug gets it into the bloodstream faster and injecting a drug intravenously works quickly too because it pumps the (6) _____ directly into the blood. Once there，the drug quickly reaches the gates of its destination，the brain. The entrance to this organ is guarded by the blood brain barrier，which separates blood from the nervous system to keep potentially dangerous substances out. So all drugs must have a specific chemical composition which gives them the key to unlock this barrier and pass through. Once inside，drugs start to（7）_____ with the brain's normal functioning by targeting its web of neurons and synapses.

inhale［ɪnˈheɪl］	*v*. to draw（breath）into the lungs；breathe in 吸入
bloodstream［ˈblʌdstriːm］	*n*. the flow of blood through the vessels of a living body 血流
intravenously［ˌɪntrəˈviːnəslɪ］	*adv*. within or administered into a vein 静脉注射地
synapse［ˈsaɪnæps］	*n*. the junction between two neurons（神经元的）突触

2. **Read the following passage and answer these questions.**

（1）What is drug safety?

_____

（2）How important is the information received from patients and healthcare providers?

_____

（3）What is clinical trial?

_____

_____

Passage A

Pharmacovigilance

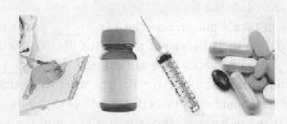

　　Pharmacovigilance，also known as drug safety，is the pharmacological science relating to the collection，detection，assessment，monitoring，and prevention of adverse effects（AE）with pharmaceutical products. Pharmacovigilance heavily focuses on adverse drug reactions（ADRs），which are defined as any response to a drug which is noxious and unintended，including lack of efficacy. Medication errors such as overdose，and misuse and abuse of a drug as well as drug exposure during pregnancy and breastfeeding，are also of interest，even without an adverse event，because they may result in an adverse drug reaction.

Information received from patients and healthcare providers via pharmacovigilance agreements, as well as other sources such as the medical literature, plays a critical role in providing the data necessary for pharmacovigilance to take place. In fact, in order to market or to test a pharmaceutical product in most countries, adverse event data received by the license holder (usually a pharmaceutical company) must be submitted to the local drug regulatory authority.

Ultimately, pharmacovigilance is concerned with identifying the hazards associated with pharmaceutical products and with minimizing the risk of any harm that may come to patients. Companies must conduct a comprehensive drug safety and pharmacovigilance audit to assess their compliance with worldwide laws, regulations, and guidance.

Some Terms Commonly Used in Drug Safety

- *Adverse drug reaction* is a side effect (non-intended reaction to the drug) occurring with a drug where a positive (direct) causal relationship between the event and the drug is thought, or has been proven, to exist.
- *Causal relationship* is said to exist when a drug is thought to have caused or contributed to the occurrence of an adverse drug reaction.
- *Clinical trial* (or study) refers to an organized program to determine the safety and/or efficacy of a drug (or drugs) in patients. The design of a clinical trial will depend on the drug and the phase of its development.
- *Control group* is a group (or cohort) of individual patients that is used as a standard of comparison within a clinical trial. The control group may be taking a placebo (where no active drug is given) or where a different active drug is given as a comparator.
- *Harm* is the nature and extent of the actual damage that could be or has been caused.
- *Implied causality* refers to spontaneously reported AE cases where the causality is always presumed to be positive unless the reporter states otherwise.
- *Individual Case Study Report* is an adverse event report for an individual patient.
- *Risk factor* is an attribute of a patient that may predispose, or increase the risk, of that patient developing an event that may or may not be drug-related. For instance, obesity is considered a risk factor for a number of different diseases and, potentially, ADRs. Others would be high blood pressure, diabetes, possessing a specific mutated gene.
- *Signal* is a new safety finding within safety data that requires further investigation. There are three categories of signals: *confirmed signals* where the data indicate that there is a causal relationship between the drug

and the AE; *refuted*（or false）*signals* where after investigation the data indicate that no causal relationship exists; and *unconfirmed signals* which require further investigation（more data）such as the conducting of a post-marketing trial to study the issue.

pharmacovigilance [ˌfɑːməkəˈvɪdʒɪləns]	*n.* a state of heightened awareness, monitoring and reporting of potentially adverse pharmacologic events 药品安全,药物警戒
noxious [ˈnɒkʃəs]	*adj.* poisonous or harmful 有毒的
hazard [ˈhæzəd]	*n.* a thing that can be dangerous or cause damage 危险,危害
comparator [kəmˈpærətə(r)]	*n.* any instruments used for making comparisons 比较仪,比测器
causality [kɔːˈzæləti]	*n.* the principle of or relationship between cause and effect 因果关系;因果性
spontaneously [spɒnˈteɪnɪəsli]	*adv.* self-generated, of one's own free will 不由自主地
predispose [ˌpriːdɪˈspəʊz]	*v.* to make sb likely to suffer from a particular illness or condition 使易于患(某种病);容易诱发
confirmed [kənˈfɜːmd]	*adj.* having been found or shown to be true or definite 证实的

3. **Match each of the terms listed below with the numbered definition. Write the letter in the space provided.**

A. noxious	E. causality	I. efficacy
B. hazard	F. adverse	J. predispose
C. prescription	G. monitor	K. confirmed
D. assessment	H. compliance	L. relentless

（1）_____ : not likely to produce a good result

（2）_____ : proved and therefore known to be true or accurate

（3）_____ : to regularly check sth or watch sb in order to find out what is happening

（4）_____ : the relationship of cause and effect

(5) _____ : a piece of paper that a doctor gives which says what medication you need

(6) _____ : effectiveness of something and its ability to do what it is supposed to

(7) _____ : the act of following or obeying something, like a law, treaty, or agreement

(8) _____ : existing or occurring without interruption or end

(9) _____ : to incline or make sb susceptible to something beforehand

(10) _____ : a consideration of sb or sth and a judgment about them

(11) _____ : poisonous or very harmful

(12) _____ : something which could be dangerous to you, your health, etc.

IV. Critical Reading — Further Reading on Medication Concerns

1. Shocking Drug Side Effects

Read the following passage and complete the exercises that follow.

A. Fill in the blanks to complete the table.

Drug	Side effects
Sleep medication	It might cause (1) _____ . People might experience memory (2) _____ after taking the sleeping pills. The drugs can (3) _____ in the body until the next morning, (4) _____ your ability to drive or do other tasks requiring (5) _____ .
Weight-loss drug	It might cause (6) _____ . People who take the drug might suffer from (7) _____ . It also (8) _____ the absorption of fat-soluble vitamins such as vitamin A, D, E, and K. Clinical trials revealed that some people had trouble (9) _____ during the first year of use of weight-loss drug, and some had other symptoms, such as (10) _____ .

B. Judge whether the following statements are true (T) or false (F).

_____ (1) The side effects of drug only cover a short and acceptable list as we get from the TV ads.

_____ (2) Medication could affect people in different ways, so talk with the doctor for consultation before you take them.

_____ (3) The consequence of sleeping pills is just to help you get to sleep.

_____ (4) Orlistat works as a kind of drug which is used to help lose weight by blocking fat absorption, and it's safe and side-effect free.

_____ (5) Drugs and pills come with the risks and inconveniences, and sometimes they outweigh their benefits in helping people.

Passage B

Shocking Drug Side Effects

Listening to the long and scary list of possible side effects in TV ads for drugs — uncontrollable bowel movements, cancer, even death — can make you want to swear off most pharmaceuticals for good. Well, that's just the tip of the iceberg. There are lots of shocking potential drug side effects that you won't hear about in ads; you'll have to read the fine print that comes with your prescription. As we've reported before, reading those package inserts will tell you, for example, that topical bimatoprost(药名,比马前列素) can help you grow longer, fuller eyelashes, but could also turn your eyes a darker shade of brown.

Other drug side effects may be less dramatic, but they're still important to know, so we've put together a list. But it isn't comprehensive; all of the drugs can cause problems other than the ones we mention. Also, keep in mind that medications affect people in different ways, so talk with your doctor if you experience symptoms after starting a drug, even if they're not listed on the package insert. And never stop taking any medication without talking to your doctor first, because that could cause other health problems.

Sleep Disorder

Caused by: Some sleep medications, including eszopiclone(药名,右佐匹克隆), ramelteon(药名,雷美替胺), and zolpidem(药名,唑吡坦).

What happens: In addition to eating, making calls, and driving — all while sleeping — some people taking these drugs have experienced memory lapses and hallucinations. Also, the drugs can linger in the body until the next morning, affecting your ability to drive or do other tasks requiring alertness. In 2013, the Food and Drug Administration reported that it had received about 700 reports of people whose driving ability was impaired or who were in an auto accident after taking the sleep drug zolpidem. As a result of those reports and data from clinical trials, drugmakers were told to cut in half the recommended dose of zolpidem in these drugs and warn people who use the extended-release version(Ambien CR) not to drive at all the day after taking it. The FDA is looking into whether similar changes are warranted for other sleep drugs. Women are especially at risk for side effects because the drugs leave their system slower than in men.

What to do: If nondrug remedies don't work for your sleep problems, you could try an over-the-counter drug that contains diphenhydramine(苯海拉明) occasionally. Next-day drowsiness can occur, so be careful when driving. Exceeding the recommended dose or mixing sleep drugs with other medications or alcohol can increase the risk of side effects.

Uncontrollable Bowel Movements

Caused by: The weight-loss drug Orlistat(药名,奥利司他), the active ingredient in the OTC drug alli(爱丽减肥胶囊), and the prescription drug Xenical(减肥

药,罗氏鲜).

What happens: Orlistat works by blocking fat absorption, which means that your body has to do something with the dietary fat it's unable to use. Virtually everyone who takes Orlistat has some diarrhea. It also hinders the absorption of fat-soluble vitamins such as vitamin A, D, E, and K. In clinical trials of Xenical, which is twice as strong as Alli, 8 percent of people had trouble controlling their bowels during the first year of use, and up to 27 percent had other symptoms, such as underwear staining and gas. And Xenical includes a warning regarding reported cases of pancreatitis (inflammation of the pancreas).

What to do: Our medical experts believe the risks and inconveniences of Orlistat vastly outweigh its benefits in helping people lose weight. You're going to be better off using proven (and non-underwear-staining) weight-loss methods such as exercising more often and eating less.

bowel [ˈbaʊəl]	*n*. the intestine 肠道
topical [ˈtɒpɪkəl]	*adj*. connected with, or put directly on, a part of the body (身体)局部的,表面的
lapse [læps]	*n*. a break in the continuity of sth 终止或失效
hallucination [həˌluːsɪˈneɪʃən]	*n*. an illusion of perceiving sth that does not really exist 幻觉,错觉
linger [ˈlɪŋɡə(r)]	*v*. to continue to exist for longer than expected 继续存留
alertness [əˈlɜːtnɪs]	*n*. the process of paying close and continuous attention 警觉,机敏
remedy [ˈremɪdɪ]	*n*. a medication or treatment that cures a disease or disorder or relieves its symptoms 治疗;疗法
drowsiness [ˈdraʊzɪnɪs]	*n*. a very sleepy state 困倦,嗜睡
pancreatitis [ˌpænkrɪəˈtaɪtɪs]	*n*. the inflammation of pancreas 胰腺炎

2. **Q & A on the Regulation on Drug Safety.**
   Read the following passage to complete the notes, and then check your understanding.

This regulation is for:	(1)_____ engaged in research, production, (2)_____, use, or drug administration in the People's Republic of China.
This law protects:	The State develops both modern and traditional medicines to fully play their role in the prevention and treatment of diseases and the maintenance of health. The State protects the resources of (3)_____ crude drugs and encourages the (4)_____ of Chinese crude drugs.
Developing new drugs:	the State encourages research and development of new drugs and protects the (5)_____ of citizens, legal bodies and other institutions engaged in this field of endeavor.
Drug safety:	(6)_____ established or designated by the drug regulatory departments shall undertake the responsibility for drug testing required for conducting drug (7)_____ and controlling drug quality in accordance with the law.
Requirements to import drug:	Drugs shall be imported via the ports where drug importation is (8)_____, and be registered by the drug importers with the local drug regulatory departments for the record. The (9)_____ shall release the drugs on the basis of the Drug Import Note issued by the said departments, and may not release those drugs for which no Drug Import Note is (10)_____.

Passage C

Q & A on the Regulation on Drug Safety

As a special commodity, drugs are substances that bear on the people's health and life. Drug regulation is the use of government regulation in the pharmaceutical field, the core of which is to ensure the safety of drugs, but we should take other basic goals such as availability, quality assurance, and reasonable use into consideration. Therefore, at the beginning of the new semester, the teacher asked the freshmen from the School of Pharmacy to get acquainted with the relevant legal issues about drug safety. Here is a medical student and his teacher discussing regulations on drug safety.

Student: Hello! I am quite interested in drug safety, could I ask you a few questions about it?

Teacher: Sure. What aspects would you like to learn?

Student: I'd like to know why should the Regulation on Drug Safety be made?

Teacher: According to Article 1 of Regulation on Drug Safety, this law is enacted to strengthen drug administration, ensure the quality and safety of drugs for people, protect people's health and safeguard their legitimate rights and interests in the use of drugs.

Student: To whom is this regulation applying?

Teacher: According to Article 2, all institutions and individuals engaged in research, production, distribution, use, or drug administration in the People's Republic of China shall abide by this law.

Student: Is every drug protected under this law?

Teacher: According to Article 3, the State develops both modern and traditional medicines to fully play their role in the prevention and treatment of diseases and the maintenance of health. The State protects the resources of natural crude drugs and encourages the cultivation of Chinese crude drugs.

Student: If I want to develop new drugs, could I get any support?

Teacher: According to Article 4, the State encourages research and development of new drugs and protects the legitimate rights and interests of citizens, legal bodies and other institutions engaged in this field of endeavor.

Student: How can we know if a drug is safe or not?

Teacher: According to Article 6, the drug testing institutes established or designated by the drug regulatory departments shall undertake the responsibility for drug testing required for conducting drug review and approval and controlling drug quality in accordance with the law.

Student: If I want to establish a drug factory, what are the qualifications should it have?

Teacher: According to Article 8, a drug manufacturer to be established must meet the following requirements:

(1) Having legally qualified pharmaceutical and technical personnel;

(2) Having the premises, facilities, and hygienic environment required for drug manufacturing;

(3) Having the facilities and personnel capable of quality control and testing of the drugs to be produced, as well as the necessary instruments and equipment;

(4) Having rules and regulations to ensure the quality of drugs.

Student: What are the requirements to import drug?

Teacher: According to Article 40, drugs shall be imported via the ports where drug importation is permitted, and be registered by the drug importers with the local drug regulatory departments for the record. The customs shall release the drugs on the basis of the Drug Import Note issued by the said departments, and may not release those drugs for which no Drug Import Note is issued.

The drug regulatory department in the place where the port is located shall notify the drug testing institution to conduct sampling and testing of the drugs to be imported according to the regulations of the drug regulatory department under the State Council, and sampling fees shall be charged in accordance with the provisions of the second paragraph of Article 41 of this Law.

The ports where drugs may be imported shall be proposed by the drug regulatory department under the State Council together with the General Administration of Customs and submitted to the State Council for approval.

Student：What will happen to the drugs which is not qualified any more?

Teacher：According to Article 42，the drug regulatory department under the State Council of the shall organize investigations of the drugs to the production or importation of which it has granted approval; it shall withdraw the approval number or Import Drug License issued to drugs with uncertain therapeutic efficacy，serious adverse reaction，or other factors harmful to human health.

No drugs whose approval numbers or import drug licenses have been withdrawn may be produced，distributed or used. Those already produced or imported shall be destroyed or disposed of under the supervision of the local drug regulatory department.

Student：How can we tell if a drug is a counterfeit drug?

Teacher：According to Article 48，production (including dispensing，the same below) and distribution of counterfeit drugs are prohibited.

A drug is a counterfeit drug in any of the following cases：

（1）The ingredients in the drug are different from those specified by the national drug standards;

（2）A non-drug substance is simulated as a drug or one drug is simulated as another.

A drug shall be treated as a counterfeit drug in any of the following cases：

（1）Its use is prohibited by the regulations of the drug regulatory department under the State Council;

（2）It is produced or imported without approval，or marketed without being tested，as required by this Law;

（3）It is deteriorated;

（4）It is contaminated;

（5）It is produced by using drug substances without approval number as required by this Law;

（6）The indications or functions indicated are beyond the specified scope.

Student：What kind of drug is not allowed to sell?

Teacher：According to Article 49，production and distribution of substandard drugs are prohibited. A drug with content not up to the national drug standards is a substandard drug. A drug shall be treated as substandard drug in any of the following cases：

（1）The date of expiry is not indicated or is altered;

（2）The batch number is not indicated or is altered;

（3）It is beyond the date of expiry;

（4）No approval is obtained for the immediate packaging material or container;

(5) Colorants, preservatives, spices, flavorings or other excipients are added without authorization;

(6) Other cases where the drug standards are not conformed.

Student: That is all I need to know, thanks a lot!

Teacher: You are welcome!

crude [kruːd]	*adj*. in its natural state, before it has been treated with chemicals 天然的；自然的
counterfeit [ˈkaʊntəfɪt]	*adj*. made to look exactly like sth in order to trick people into thinking that they are getting the real thing 伪造的；仿造的；假冒的
colorant [ˈkʌlərənt]	*n*. a substance that is used to put colour in sth, especially a person's hair 着色剂；染色剂
preservative [prɪˈzɜːvətɪv]	*n*. a substance used to prevent food or wood from decaying 防腐剂；保护剂
excipient [ekˈsɪpiənt]	*n*. an inactive substance that serves as the vehicle or medium for a drug or other active substance（用作药物载体的）赋形剂
conform [kənˈfɔːm]	*v*. to obey a rule, law, etc. 遵守，遵从，服从（规则、法律等）

3. Lexical chunks and sentence rewriting

A. Substitute the underlined parts with the words or expressions you have learned.

(1) Pharmacovigilance <u>heavily focuses on</u> adverse drug reactions, or ADRs, which are defined as any response to a drug ... (Passage A)

Answer:

Pharmacovigilance _____ adverse drug reactions, or ADRs, which are defined as any response to a drug ...

(2) Pharmacovigilance is concerned with identifying the hazards <u>associated with</u> pharmaceutical products and with <u>minimizing</u> the risk of any harm that may come to patients. (Passage A)

Answer:

Pharmacovigilance is concerned with identifying the hazards _____ pharmaceutical products and with _____ the risk of any harm that may come to patients.

(3) The design of a clinical trial will <u>depend on</u> the drug and the phase of its development. (Passage A)

Answer:

The design of a clinical trial will _____ the drug and the phase of its development.

(4) Also, the drugs can <u>linger in</u> the body until the next morning, affecting your

ability to drive or do other tasks requiring alertness. (Passage B)

Answer：

Also，the drugs can _____ the body until the next morning，affecting your ability to drive or do other tasks requiring alertness.

(5) Exceeding the recommended dose or mixing sleep drugs with other medications or alcohol can increase the risk of side effects. (Passage B)

Answer：

_____ the recommended dose or mixing sleep drugs with other medications or alcohol can increase the risk of side effects.

(6) Our medical experts believe the risks and inconveniences of orlistat vastly outweigh its benefits in helping people lose weight. (Passage B)

Answer：

Our medical experts believe the risks and inconveniences of orlistat vastly _____ its benefits in helping people lose weight.

(7) The ports where drugs may be imported shall be proposed by the drug regulatory department under the State Council together with the General Administration of Customs and submitted to the State Council for approval. (Passage C)

Answer：

The ports where drugs may be imported shall be _____ by the drug regulatory department under the State Council together with the General Administration of Customs and submitted to the State Council for approval.

(8) It shall withdraw the approval number or Import Drug License issued to drugs with uncertain therapeutic efficacy，serious adverse reaction，or other factors harmful to human health(Passage C)

Answer：

It shall withdraw the approval number or Import Drug License issued to drugs with uncertain therapeutic efficacy，serious _____ reaction，or other factors harmful to human health.

(9) It is contaminated. (Passage C)

Answer：

It is _____ .

B. Rewrite the following sentences using the academic expressions you have learned in the articles.

(1) Ultimately，pharmacovigilance is concerned with identifying the hazards associated with pharmaceutical products and with minimizing the risk of any harm that may come to patients. (Passage A)

Lexical chunks：_____

Sentence rewriting：_____

_____

(2) Also，the drugs can linger in the body until the next morning，affecting your ability to drive or do other tasks requiring alertness. (Passage B)

Lexical chunks：_____

Sentence rewriting: _____

(3) It also hinders the absorption of fat-soluble vitamins such as vitamin A, D, E, and K. (passage B)
  Lexical chunks: _____
  Sentence rewriting: _____
  _____

(4) In 2013, the Food and Drug Administration reported that it had received about 700 reports of people whose driving ability was impaired or who were in an auto accident after taking the sleep drug zolpidem. (Passage B)
  Lexical chunks: _____
  Sentence rewriting: _____
  _____

(5) When a new Drug has gone through clinical trials and passed the evaluation, a New Drug Certificate shall be issued upon approval by the drug regulatory by department under the State Council. (Passage C)
  Lexical chunks: _____
  Sentence rewriting: _____
  _____

4. **Bilingual translation**

   Put the following into Chinese or vice versa.

   A. English-Chinese translation

   Learn the following useful expressions by translating the sentences selected from the passage.

   (1) as a result 结果,因此

   Excerpt:

   As a result of those reports and data from clinical trials, drugmakers were told to cut in half the recommended dose of zolpidem in these drugs and warn people who use the extended-release version (Ambien CR) not to drive at all the day after taking it.

   Translation:

   _____
   _____

   (2) keep in mind 挂心,铭记于心

   Excerpt:

   Also, keep in mind that medications affect people in different ways, so talk with your doctor if you experience symptoms after starting a drug, even if they're not listed on the package insert.

   Translation:

   _____
   _____

   (3) better off 情况好转

   Excerpt:

You're going to be better off using proven weight-loss methods such as exercising more often and eating less.

Translation：

_____

_____

（4）be warranted for 被需要的

Excerpt：

The FDA is looking into whether similar changes are warranted for other sleep drugs.

Translation：

_____

_____

（5）outweigh 超过

Excerpt：

Our medical experts believe the risks and inconveniences of Orlistat vastly outweigh its benefits in helping people lose weight.

Translation：

_____

_____

（6）virtually 几乎

Excerpt：

Virtually everyone who takes Orlistat has some diarrhea.

Translation：

_____

_____

（7）hinder 阻碍，妨碍

Excerpt：

It also hinders the absorption of fat-soluble vitamins such as vitamin A，D，E，and K.

Translation：

_____

_____

B. Chinese-English translation

Put the Chinese paragraph into English.

第五十一条　药品生产企业、药品经营企业和医疗机构直接接触药品的工作人员，必须每年进行健康检查。患有传染病或者其他可能污染药品的疾病的人员，不得从事直接接触药品的工作。

_____

_____

_____

_____

_____
_____
_____

V. Speaking-out   Knowledge About Medicine

1. Read and say

Look at the pictures and the information on them. Work in pairs and discuss the information with your partner. Note down your key points in the blanks.

What Is the Name of My Medicine, and How Should I Take It?

Get the Facts

Ask your pharmacist to explain the instructions on your prescription label.

1

Did You Know?

60% of patients misunderstand the instructions for how to take their medicines.

Q _____
Q _____
Q _____
Q _____
Q _____
Q _____
Q _____
Q _____

What Information Do You Need To Know About the Other Medicines That I Am Taking?

2 **Write It Down**

Keep a medicine list with the name, dose, and schedule of all the medications, vitamins, and herbal products you take. Share it with your pharmacist or doctor.

Did You Know?

50% of all hospital medication errors happen because patients have not told their doctor or pharmacist about the medications they are taking.

Q _____
Q _____
Q _____
Q _____
Q _____
Q _____
Q _____
Q _____

When Should I Take This Medication?

Make It Work

The time of day you take your medicine can affect how well it works. Ask your pharmacist about what time to take your medicine.

3

Did You Know?

Taking certain blood pressure medicines at night may help control blood pressure better, reducing the risk of heart attack or stroke.

Q _____
Q _____
Q _____
Q _____
Q _____
Q _____
Q _____
Q _____

What Are the Common Side Effects of This Medicine?

4 **Know Your Risks**
Check out SafeMedication.com for potential side effects and what to do if they occur.

Did You Know?

290,000 pharmacists in the U.S. have the education and training to help you with your medicines.

Improving your English at home

- **Record yourself.** When you're by your lonesome，you have no reason to be nervous. You can let your brain flow freely — so record yourself now! Your English is going to be at its best. Find a book on tape or a clip online that you can mimic.
- **Read aloud.** If your hands are full or you don't have a recording device，simply read aloud — ideally，every day for at least 15 or 20 minutes.
- **Listen to MP3s，podcasts，and the news.** Scientific American，CBC，BBC and Australia's ABC Radio are great MP3s to get started with.
- **Listen to music，too.** Make sure you actively try to understand the song. Search the lyrics and sing along.
- **Watch TV and movies.** An integral part of speaking is hearing or listening. Because of this，the easiest way to involve yourself in a conversation without actually having one is to watch English TV and movies.
- **Narrate your world.** As you go about your day-to-day，talk to yourself. What are you doing? What are you feeling? What do you see，taste，smell，hear? What are you touching? What are you thinking? The possibilities are limitless.

Useful tips to start a good conversation：

- Make the person feel like his thoughts are important. If he begins to talk about a subject，ask more questions about it instead of talking about something that you really want to talk about.
- Use the person's name once or twice after you learn it.
- If the person talks first，nod intently to show that you're listening.
- If you realize that you've been asking too many questions，make a joke about it. Say，"Sorry — the interview is over，" and move on to talking about something else.
- Ask the person about his hobbies or interests，not about his dreams and desires.
- Talk about something fun. Don't ask the person what he thinks about the latest tragedy on the news or how much he's had to work overtime recently. Make the person enjoy the subject of the conversation as well as the conversation itself.
- Make sure that you're sharing，too. Ideally，you and the other person should share the same amount.

---

2. **Watch and act**

   Watch a video clip. Fill in the blanks and then act out the speech in class.

   So you go to the doctor and get some tests.

   The doctor （1）_____ that you have high cholesterol and you would benefit from medication to treat it.

So you get a (2) _____ .

You have some confidence, your physician has some confidence that this is going to work. The company that invented it did a lot of studies, (3) _____ it to the FDA. They studied it very carefully, (4) _____ , they (5) _____ it. They have a rough idea of how it works; they have a rough idea of what the side effects are. It should be OK.

You have a little more of a conversation with your physician and the physician is a little worried because you've been blue, you haven't felt like yourself, you haven't been able to enjoy things in life quite as much as you usually do.

Your physician says, "You know, I think you have some (6) _____ . I'm going to have to give you another pill."

So now we're talking about two medications.

This pill also — millions of people have taken it, the company did studies, the FDA looked at it — all good. Think things should go OK.

Well, wait a minute. How much have we studied these two together? Well, it's very hard to do that. In fact, it's not (7) _____ done.

We totally depend on what we call "(8) _____ surveillance", after the drugs hit the market. How can we figure out if bad things are happening between two medications? Three? Five? Seven? Ask your favorite person who has several (9) _____ how many medication they are on.

Why do I care about this problem? I care about it deeply. I'm an informatics and data science guy and really, in my opinion, the only hope — only hope — to understand these (10) _____ is to leverage lots of different sources of data in order to figure out when drugs can be used together safely and when it's not so safe.

VI. Pros/Cons Ten Drug Safety Tips for Patients

1. **Read the following passage with ten tips attached to it. Each tip contains information given in one of the paragraphs. Identify the paragraph from which the information is derived. You may choose a paragraph more than once. Each paragraph is marked with a letter.**

_____ (1) Not sure your online pharmacy is legitimate? Visit Legitscript to check that it is a legitimate pharmacy.

_____ (2) Ask your doctor to see packaging for your medication. Does the packaging look genuine to you?

_____ (3) Be wary of scam artists online who try to sell you discount prescription cards or ask for too much personal information.

_____ (4) Don't buy prescription drugs from pharmacy websites that do not require prescriptions!

_____ （5）During flu season, beware of too-good-to-be-true flu cures and treatments. They are probably fake.

_____ （6）Question natural remedies. Don't believe that a "natural" remedy is a genuine treatment. It may be a dangerous unapproved pharmaceutical that has skirted the FDA approval process.

_____ （7）Check the label on your prescription.

_____ （8）Closely examine the appearance of your medication.

_____ （9）Pay attention to changes in the taste of your pills.

_____ （10）Do not ignore your symptoms if you experience side effects from a new dose of your prescription.

A) Are the pills cracked or chipped? Has the pill color changed? Does it appear a shade different from earlier prescriptions? Manufacturers of both name-brand and generic drugs take great pains to produce drugs of uniform and standardized appearance. Every change to a drug's appearance must go through an approval process, so if the pills look different, they are probably fake.

B) Any site that does not need a prescription is likely selling fake drugs. If you visit an online pharmacy to purchase your medication, they should require the submission of a copy of your prescription in digital or fax form. If they instead tell you they do not need it, or simply have you fill out a form or respond to questions, be suspicious. If they fail to require a prescription, it is likely they have no compunction about selling you cheaply-made counterfeits.

C) When you buy prescriptions at a pharmacy, you can always ask the pharmacist to show you the bottle your prescription came in. But what if you are being treated with medication at your doctor's office? Before you ingest medication at a doctor's office or clinic, request to see the packaging the drugs came in, and be on the lookout for accurate labeling, the condition of the package, and the language of the labeling. All prescriptions approved for sale in the US should have product descriptions in English.

D) Is label crooked? Does it look different than previous prescriptions of the same drug? Are the instructions in English? Does the packaging look clean and correctly sealed? When comparing packaging, look for differences in paper, printing, color, and fonts (i.e. is it the same size, raised print, embossed, etc.). If you notice changes, do not take the drugs, and show the packaging to your doctor.

E) Legitscript provides a free online assessment tool for consumers to check the legitimacy of an Internet pharmacy. They do this by verifying that the website in question adheres to all applicable laws and regulations. They also provide a frequently updated list of sites to avoid, and champion efforts to take down fake online pharmacies.

F) Every year, colds, influenza and other seasonal illnesses make their way across the United States. Health practitioners try to encourage vaccination, but drug counterfeiters see these epidemics as a money-making opportunity. Before deciding to try a flu treatment you see advertised online or in advertisements, ask your doctor about whether he/she has heard of it. If not, don't take a chance with a fly-by-night cure.

G) Does the drug taste different? If your drugs do not seem to have the same taste or if you feel different than usual, immediately write down your symptoms and contact your doctor and pharmacist.

H) Genuine patient prescription assistance programs never ask for money for their services.

I) Did you experience any adverse effects, or did treatment not work at all? Is there anything unusual in your body's reaction compared to previous experiences, such as a stomachache or headache? This could be a sign that the drug you took contained a different compound than it was supposed to or did not contain any genuine drug at all.

J) Every year, the FDA sends warnings about purportedly herbal remedies that instead contain dangerous or unapproved pharmaceutical ingredients. Since these remedies are not classified as pharmaceuticals, their manufacturers can skip the FDA approval process by calling them "supplements". In so doing, they dodge oversight that is applied to medication. Natural remedies may be just what they say they are, or they may contain dangerous drugs not approved for US sale. Only buy natural remedies from verified sources that clearly state their ingredients. Also watch out for natural remedies that make medical claims that can't be substantiated.

2. **Read the following statements. Decide to what extent you agree or disagree with each statement, and write your own pros or cons in the box, then set out your rational viewpoint and the reasons.**

(1) Drugs are available online today, and it's safe and convenient to buy your prescriptions from an online pharmacy.

(2) Advertised drugs usually get its approval from authorities, and it's safe to buy them from the pharmacy without a doctor's prescription.

Pros	Cons

VII. Outcome　Sentence Analysis and Essay Writing

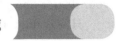

1. Sentence-structure analysis

Analyze the following sentences and draw a tree-structure.

(1) Medication errors such as overdose, and misuse and abuse of a drug as well as drug exposure during pregnancy and breastfeeding, are also of interest, even without an adverse event, because they may result in an adverse drug reaction.

(2) As we've reported before, reading those package inserts will tell you, for example, that topical bimatoprost can help you grow longer, fuller eyelashes, but could also turn your eyes a darker shade of brown.

(3) In 2013, the Food and Drug Administration reported that it had received about 700 reports of people whose driving ability was impaired or who were in an auto accident after taking the sleep drug zolpidem.

(4) Drug regulation is the use of government regulation in the pharmaceutical field, the core of which is to ensure the safety of drugs, but we should take other basic goals such as availability, quality assurance, reasonable use into consideration.

(5) The drug testing institutes established or designated by the drug regulatory departments shall undertake the responsibility for drug testing required for conducting drug review and approval and controlling drug quality in accordance with the law.

2. Essay writing

Everyone has a role to play in medication safety. Write a public letter to strengthen people's awareness of the importance of drug safety. In your letter, you should tell people why they need to do this and what they can do.

_____

_____

_____

_____

_____

_____

_____

_____

_____

_____

_____

_____

_____

_____

Unit 1 Unit 2 Unit 3 Unit 4 Unit 5 Unit 6 Unit 7 Unit 8

图书在版编目(CIP)数据

医学人文英语. 下册/杨劲松,徐琴,刘娅主编. —3 版. —上海：复旦大学出版社, 2024.1
医学人文英语系列教材 / 杨劲松总主编
ISBN 978-7-309-16558-6

Ⅰ.①医⋯　Ⅱ.①杨⋯ ②徐⋯ ③刘⋯　Ⅲ.①医学-人文科学-英语-医学院校-教材　Ⅳ.①R

中国版本图书馆 CIP 数据核字(2022)第 201018 号

医学人文英语(下册)第三版
杨劲松　徐　琴　刘　娅　主编
责任编辑/江黎涵　任　战

复旦大学出版社有限公司出版发行
上海市国权路 579 号　邮编：200433
网址：fupnet@ fudanpress.com　http://www.fudanpress.com
门市零售：86-21-65102580　　团体订购：86-21-65104505
出版部电话：86-21-65642845
上海丽佳制版印刷有限公司

开本 787 毫米×1092 毫米　1/16　印张 15　字数 332 千字
2024 年 1 月第 3 版第 1 次印刷
印数 1—11 000

ISBN 978-7-309-16558-6/R · 2007
定价：69.00 元